QIGONG THROUGH THE SEASONS

QIGONG THROUGH THE SEASONS

How to Stay Healthy All Year Long
with Qigong, Meditation, Diet, and Herbs

RONALD H. DAVIS

FOREWORD BY KENNETH COHEN

ILLUSTRATIONS BY PAMM DAVIS

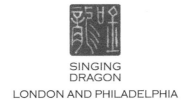

SINGING
DRAGON
LONDON AND PHILADELPHIA

First published in 2015
by Singing Dragon
an imprint of Jessica Kingsley Publishers
73 Collier Street
London N1 9BE, UK
and
400 Market Street, Suite 400
Philadelphia, PA 19106, USA

www.singingdragon.com

Library of Congress Cataloging in Publication Data
Davis, Ronald H.
Qigong through the seasons : how to stay healthy all year with qigong, meditation, diet and herbs / Ronald H. Davis.
pages cm
Includes bibliographical references and index.
ISBN 978-1-84819-238-6 (alk. paper)
1. Qi gong. 2. Health. I. Title.
RA781.8.D39 2015
613.7'1489--dc23
2014030112

British Library Cataloguing in Publication Data
A CIP catalogue record for this book is available from the British Library

ISBN 978 1 84819 238 6
eISBN 978 0 85701 185 5

Printed and bound in Great Britain

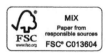

To Pamm, without whom I would not be the man I am.

Contents

FOREWORD

The ancient Taoist classic, Zhuang Zi, tells the story of a man standing at the edge of a raging river. Suddenly the man jumps into the torrent, lets the water carry him a bit, and then just as effortlessly climbs ashore. Stuffy old Confucius, watching the scene and probably offended by the man's lack of caution and unconventional behavior, asks him how he managed not to drown. The man replies, "I just go in with a swirl, come out with a whirl and follow the flow of the water, not thinking of myself."

The only changeless thing in the world is change itself. Philosophers in all times and places have agreed with this concept. The Greek philosopher Heraclitus said: "All things flow; you can't step twice into the same river." Yet, many people, faced with change and the stress of adapting to changing circumstances, retreat into rigidity. They develop an unchanging strategy, part physical, part mental, to avoid novelty. No matter what life presents them they have a similar response, always an angry word or always a cheerful, yet artificial, smile. This habit of bracing against change rather than flowing with it tends to increase with age. Thus, as the founder of Taoism, Lao Zi, reminds us in his fourth century BCE classic, the *Dao De Jing*, the old tree, stiff and brittle, easily breaks. The sap of life, what the Chinese call qi, no longer flows as strongly or smoothly. "Suppleness is the companion of life; rigidity is the companion of death," Lao Zi advises.

Today, with the quick pace of life and the demands of ever-accelerating technology, the challenge of creative and flexible adaptation is greater than ever. In the 1930s endocrinologist Hans Selye defined stress as a non-specific response to the demands of change; when the response is poor—such as rising blood pressure during a traffic jam or a weakened immune system because of stage fright—the result may be disease. Not surprisingly, in the United States

40 million people suffer from anxiety disorders and at least 75 percent of all visits to health care providers are for stress-related illnesses. The good news is that something can be done about this. But I believe that the answer will not come solely from our modern medical system but rather from the wisdom of ancient cultures, such as China, that remind us of the principles of self-care and planet-care that are at the root of our humanity.

We cannot survive by using nature, but only by listening to nature and behaving in accordance with what we "hear." Nature and the cycles of nature are still the primary regulators of our biological rhythms. The light of sunrise and sunset optimizes our brain's melatonin levels, encouraging restful sleep and meaningful dreams. Indoor lighting, even full-spectrum lighting, cannot accomplish this. No matter how much we isolate ourselves from the heat of summer or the cold of winter or ignore the beauty of the full moon, we still experience their tides of influence. And how sad that today many children have to be told that food does not grow on supermarket shelves or wrapped in plastic. Humanity might think that it depends on industry, but in fact we are still, all of us, completely dependent on nature to survive. It has always been so, and always will be, because we *are* nature.

And this is why the message of Ron Davis' book is so important. *Qigong Through the Seasons* is more than a book about "ancient Chinese exercises and meditations," the common definition of qigong. Rather, it is about the skills (gong) necessary to cultivate and harmonize with the energies of life (Qi). These energies change and cycle over time. Spring Qi is different from Autumn Qi, and so our diet, herbal tonics, state of mind, and level and quality of activity, must change accordingly. "Staying tuned to the rhythms of life makes beautiful music," Dr. Davis reminds us.

Dr. Davis knows these principles not only because he is well educated but, more importantly, because he lives them. He is a former Montana cowboy turned chiropractor, acupuncturist, and qigong teacher, who has benefitted personally from the therapies he recommends. He has spent enough time living outdoors to have learned the lessons of Yin and Yang, cold and heat, and humility in the face of majestic mountains and powerful thunderstorms. (Not surprisingly, the Latin word for earth, "humus," is the root of the word "humility.") The earth is a theme Dr. Davis returns to again and again, for it is the symbolic center of the four seasons and five elements or "phases."

Mother Teresa, Catholic nun and Nobel Peace Prize winner, once said, "I alone cannot change the world, but I can cast a stone across the waters to create many ripples." My hope is that this beautiful book will also create many ripples and help foster the focus and compassion so needed in our world.

Kenneth Cohen, Qigong Master and China scholar, is the winner of the Lifetime Achievement Award in Energy Medicine. He is the author of The Way of Qigong: The Art and Science of Chinese Energy Healing.

ACKNOWLEDGMENTS

The material for this book was mined from class handouts going back to the late 1980s. The feedback from students was invaluable in teaching me how to convey abstract ideas in written words. I deeply treasure the times we had together—and still have—in the qigong and *taiji* classes. And I respectfully appreciate the wisdom, humor and good-heartedness of the authentic teachers I have trained with all over the globe, from the Wudang Mountains of China to the harbors of Los Angeles; their embodiment of the qigong lifestyle is the epitome of great teaching. The text and layout of this book would be of a much lesser quality were it not for the contributions and suggestions of Mark Schlenz, wordsmith extraordinaire, and Jane Freeburg, sweet editor at large, who have led me through the hills and valleys of writing this book. The beautiful line drawings and precise graphics that are such an important part of this project come from the expressive hand and meticulous patience of Pamm Davis. Publisher Jessica Kingsley sent a wonderful message of encouragement with her first email. That initial support buoyed a listing ship more than once. The cheerful and thoughtful comments from her and her assistants, Jane Evans and Sarah Minty, have helped carry the project to completion. A thousand bows to all of you.

PREFACE

I made my way to the chiropractor's office after a sleepless night. As he watched me struggle to get onto the adjusting table, he lifted two fingers. "You know, for a college graduate," he said, "you are really stupid." The ceiling light haloed his upright fingers. "If you keep up this lifestyle," he went on, "in two years you are going to be a cripple for life." For the past five years I had been living a dream come true: being a cowboy in charge of hundreds of cattle over 50,000 acres of land in Montana's beautiful Flathead Valley. Doing hard physical work across vast tracts of forest and grasslands, working closely with horses, cattle, and dogs, living outdoors in all types of weather—contrasted sharply with my recent college years as an honor student in religious studies and comparative literature. But the party was over. Chiropractic care was the only thing that really allowed me to last as long as I did in living out my dream. But the latest in a line of horse-related injuries left me with two broken vertebrae in my neck and one in my upper back. Those debilities, on top of dealing with severe sciatica from an exploded lumbar disc for a year, convinced me it was time for a change. Dr. Marvin Harris of Great Falls, Montana, had the gumption to say, "Why don't you use your previous degree to help meet the requirements for chiropractic college?" And so I did. That was over 30 years ago.

I enthusiastically returned to college with a commitment to help others benefit from the natural healing methods of chiropractic care based on the premise that our health status depends on how well our three nervous systems are functioning. The central, peripheral, and autonomic systems make connections at the spinal articulations; dysfunction at these motor units can lead to a plethora of problems resulting from too much or too little nervous system control. My chiropractic college offered one of the first acupuncture programs in the United States, so I studied the nervous system of Western medicine and the meridian system (a network of pathways that carry Qi, vital energy, throughout the body) of Chinese medicine simultaneously.

For thousands of years the Chinese have been saying that you can influence a person's health by performing acupuncture at specific points close to the spinal joints. I can still recall my astonishment the day we were comparing the autonomic nervous system and the meridian system adjacent to the spine and realizing the two systems had close to 80 percent corroboration on assigning very specific spinal levels to certain internal organ systems. I was fascinated by the knowledge the ancient Chinese possessed without using methods of modern scientific research. For example, Chinese medicine stated thousands of years ago that acupuncture performed at the third and fourth thoracic vertebrae (my T3 was broken) can affect lung function; Western anatomical research done in the nineteenth century found nerve connections between these same spinal levels and the lungs. This and many other correlations between the two systems fired my desire to someday be able to provide both chiropractic and acupuncture as complementary arms of a natural health care practice.

It took more than a year of postgraduate study to finally earn professional licensing for both healing arts in addition to a diplomate status in acupuncture from the top national accrediting agency. From the beginning I wanted to teach people how to help themselves achieve the promise of well-being through Chinese medical care. Acupuncture, herbal medicine, and qigong comprise the three main ingredients of that medicine, so I set out to learn about qigong. Since that time I have associated with many qigong teachers from the United States, Canada, China, and Europe during the past 30 years. The journey has involved many phases of mystery, rewards, disappointments, epiphanies, and hard-core practical value. The benefits accrue and become more interesting as the journey continues. Some of those benefits concern the very foundation of well-being: a sense of being at ease in body and calm in mind, feeling that all body parts are united and harmonious in function, having a more optimistic view of life, projecting confidence and tranquility, having more energy during the day and sleeping better at night. Simple things like that—utterly precious and hard to find.

My mother worked as a Registered Nurse for over 60 years of her life. She was very happy upon hearing that I was going to chiropractic school rather than medical school; she knew the good and the bad of our dominant health care system and was appalled at how frequently iatrogenic damage occurred.

Fatal prescription drug reactions are the fourth leading cause of death in US hospitals (after cancer, heart attacks, and strokes have defeated standard hospital care). Adverse prescription drug reactions send 4.5 million Americans to the hospital every year. We now have a new medical syndrome called the "Drug Cascade," which comes about when prescription drugs cause health problems unrelated to the health condition they are prescribed to treat. Too many people are taking drugs to treat the side-effects of drugs.

Western science performs well at heroic medicine. Aggressive intervention in sudden trauma and acute disease has saved millions of lives before the illness or injury could overwhelm the body's defense system. But Western medicine has miserably failed in the area of chronic degenerative diseases that develop over a long time and involve multiple systems. And these are the problems that are becoming more important as people live longer: cancer, arthritis, dementia, diabetes, organ dysfunction, and neurologic degeneration. These complex and enduring health problems are often contingent on personal lifestyle options. For most people, what they think, do, and say has more of a long-term effect on their health than pathogens and accidents.

From the beginning of my studies I was impressed by the emphasis that Chinese medicine put on evaluating the entire context of an individual's life—the personal, social, and spiritual levels of being. The inclusive framework that puts body, mind, and Spirit in the same room with acupuncture, herbs, and qigong has had a strong pull on my desire to offer comprehensive health care to my patients. That's why I wrote this book.

I have met extraordinary practitioners of qigong and meditation during my nearly 30 years of training. Roger Jahnke provided my first inspirational experience of qigong practice. Ken Cohen epitomizes the scholar/warrior tradition of Chinese internal arts with his extraordinary abilities as healer and teacher. Liang Shouyu is known worldwide as a grandmaster and teacher of both qigong and martial arts. Eva Wong illuminates the principles of authentic qigong through her scholarly and practical translations of the classic texts from the Daoist canon. Although they come from diverse cultures and backgrounds, these remarkable individuals have at least one thing in common: the belief that a qigong practice is not just about exercise but is primarily concerned with developing a healthy, ethical, and compassionate outlook on the world.

And so it is with *Qigong Through the Seasons*. This program presents my contribution to developing better global health, sanity, and goodwill for all of humanity. "Qigong" will be used two ways in this book. First as a set of body movements, breathing patterns, and mental intentions for cultivating personal energy, and secondly as a broader term encompassing qigong exercises, meditation practice, dietary considerations, and lifestyle refinements. I am not the originator of all these exercises and meditations. Most are based on what I have learned from my teachers and have practiced for a long time. Some of the exercises have been slightly modified due to my experience of how they work and how they could best be taught. And a scant few have evolved from my own experiential practice.

I offer this book as a manual of advice and education for your personal health enhancement by way of natural therapeutics. Tested over many generations of practitioners, these traditional healing methods have been found to be safe and effective for empowering people to restore and maintain a desirable level of well-being. You should not wait until you are sick and then rely on pharmaceutical drugs, invasive diagnostic tests, or surgeries to solve the problem of why you feel unwell. Your health, your whole life, will be better if you learn to access and use the phenomenal healing energy of the natural world, which is the essence of the strategies set forth in this book. However, only use particular substances for specific remedial or therapeutic purposes in consultation with a licensed health care practitioner.

The first five chapters are presentations and explications on the principles underlying my program. A good grasp of the concepts, tenets, and theories that support the practice is essential for you to get the full benefit of *Qigong Through the Seasons*. Otherwise you cannot become fully engaged and will less likely understand what you can accomplish with the practices. It will be well worth your time to read this section before going into the practice chapters. Here's a quick summary: to live a healthy and contented life you need to live harmoniously in the present time here on planet earth; that harmony has four distinct themes.

The next four chapters present the full program for each season. The fundamental assumption for practice stands on the fact that we are inescapably part of nature and when changes occur in nature, corresponding changes will occur within us. The cycling of the four seasons functions as the basis of organic change on earth and exerts extraordinary influence on our health. Each practice chapter exists as a comprehensive program of qigong exercise, foods, herbs, and specific meditations that will help you stay healthy during that time of year.

Every major topic in these chapters could be further explored with the knowledge gained, adding to your deeper understanding of the principles and practices presented. But the most important thing for every practitioner is to practice. And keep practicing. After you have definitely noticed the benefits from having a regular personal practice throughout the year, you may want to delve deeper into the literature. The books listed in the Reference section are great resources, but practice comes first. The healthy rewards of this program relate directly to the sincerity of your practice. Every time you do qigong or meditate, you get some benefit—the more practice, the more benefits.

I sincerely hope that you, the reader, will be inspired to adopt a lifestyle of healthy self-care based on the program presented here. These practices have without a doubt improved the quality of my life. The older I become, the more I understand the importance of doing something good for your health every day. Everyone knows that everything changes. This book will show you why the most vital changes that affect your health are governed by the seasonal cycles of nature. You will learn how to have a simple—yet profound—daily practice of qigong, meditation, and a healthy diet to help you enjoy this beautiful life all year long.

Chapter 1

Qigong

Origins

Imagine you have just woken up in a mud and grass hut on the edge of a field 2000 years ago in northern China. You do not hear a motor or television set—only the sounds of wind, birds, and water running in a shallow ditch. You pull off a thin blanket of raw silk cloth and step outside into the spring sunshine. Your muscles and joints are stiff from the cold bed. As you walk to your field of millet, crisp early-morning air carries scents of fertile soil and new growth. Before bending to your daily work, you stand facing the rising sun for a few moments. Then you move your arms out to the side and slowly overhead as you gather the sun's warmth into your hands. Your tongue tip gently touches the roof of your mouth; you feel your spine opening up. As you exhale, your hands slowly come down the front of your body until they point toward the earth. You feel relaxed, yet full of the sun's energy. You repeat this movement numerous times; then stand very still and peaceful as the sun rises further into the sky. You feel a deep bond to the earth, sun, wind, and water. You just did qigong.

People were different back then. There was no digital noise, no fluorescent lighting, and no other man-made distractions in their world. Their seamless proximity to natural phenomena gave rise to an exquisite awareness of impending weather, seasonal changes, and planetary cycles that could influence their lives. They formulated strategies of ritual, prayer, and divination to deal with those forces in order to avoid calamities and promote higher standards of living. Weather was the first crucial concern. The ability to predict storms, droughts, freezes, or floods was essential to immediate survival and to cultural development. Therefore, shamans, oracles, and astrologers became vital citizens of every community.

Shamans performed an integral part in the royal court during the Zhou dynasty (1028–221 BCE). Their official duties included ceremonies, predictions, and healing sessions. These methods often featured sacred dances that created a harmonious connection between celestial forces and terrestrial events in the hope of insuring favorable weather, bountiful harvests, and successful hunting. Shamans also performed animal dances to improve their health and professional skills.

By imitating the movements of certain animals—bear, tiger, crane, monkey, and deer—they could take on the persona and power of those creatures. These animal movements have been practiced in various forms and sets from the distant past to modern times. The most famous of these sets, the Five Animal Frolics created by Hua Tuo around 150 CE, remains "one of the oldest continuously practiced healing exercise systems in the world" (Cohen 1997, p.199). Some of the Animal Frolics are part of the *Qigong Through the Seasons* practice.

Most people spent their lives doing domestic tasks such as growing and gathering food, making shelters, and raising families. But others, called sages, were deeply connected to nature in a way so elemental that it is almost incomprehensible to us in this modern age. Meditation and qigong practice performed an integral function in the sages' lives. It allowed them to achieve tranquility and extrasensory awareness. Sages could detect subtle connections between internal body systems and observable phenomena. They were the first doctors to discover how to combine medicinal herbs, acupuncture techniques, qigong exercise, and seasonal therapeutics into an effective healing system.

Some of the sages—those who were devoted to advanced practices of meditation, qigong, and healing—were able to attain such rarefied states of existence that they were called "immortals." The Yellow Emperor explains what it took to become an immortal:

> They extracted essence from nature and practiced various disciplines such as Dao-(y)in and Qi Gong, and breathing and visualization exercises, to integrate the body, mind and spirit. They remained undisturbed and thus attained extraordinary levels of accomplishment. The immortals kept their mental energies focused and harmonized their bodies with the environment. Thus they did not show conventional signs of aging and were able to live beyond biological limitations. (Ni 1995, pp.3–4)

Did the immortals live forever? No, their bodies eventually died (there is no valid record of their current existence). But they did live far longer than the "biological limitations" of most people at that time; and their exemplary life still lives in the Daoist canon. The Emperor used exaggeration to make a point: if we use qigong and meditation wisely, and live in harmony with nature, we can attain a level of longevity and wisdom ("accomplishment") that leads to the spiritual awakening of a fully realized human being.

People have always sought ways to improve their health and lengthen their lives so that they could enjoy love, companionship, and the bounties of the earth for as long as possible. Human beings exist for two reasons: 1) because the earth has enough raw materials to support carbon based physical life; and 2) because we have an encoded predilection toward compassion for all sentient beings. The earth provides the necessities to build a body, but the fundamental purpose of human life—to awaken our innate Spirit—compels us to seek harmony among all life forms. This purpose makes us different from other animals. In a very real sense, we are lords of the earth. And while the current epoch seems bent on destruction, in the long run we endeavor to preserve and enhance all earthly life, thus fulfilling our mission to awaken the Spirit. And the longer we live, the better our chance of completing that goal. Longevity has always been highly esteemed among all cultures. Over the course of civilization, people have developed innumerable methods to attain better health, expand awareness, and prolong life.

Chinese history contains hundreds of exercise techniques that came to be called qigong, such as *Yang Sheng* (Nurturing Life), *Tu Na* (Exhalation and Inhalation), *Xing Qi* (Circulating Qi), *Jing Zuo* (Sitting Meditation), and *Dao Yin* (Guiding and Conducting). The word "qigong" first appeared in a text by the Daoist master Xu Sun during the Jin dynasty (265–420 CE), but it was not used extensively until the early twentieth century. The term was officially endorsed in 1955 with the opening of the Tangshan Qigong Sanitarium in Hebei province (Tianjun and Chen 2010).

Qigong Through the Seasons presents a comprehensive program for nurturing your life by using qigong, meditation, and diet, while maintaining an insightful awareness of nature in all of its manifestations. This physical, mental, and spiritual relationship with nature becomes more important to our health as our culture becomes increasingly embedded in a world of man-made technologies and drifts away from living a life based on the energy flows and cyclical changes of the natural world. Humans cannot supersede nature. We see the ultimate power of nature whenever fierce storms or earthquakes shut down lines of communication and leave us without electricity and computers. We need to relearn how to access the essence of nature, how to keep our mental energies focused, and how to harmonize our bodies with the environment. If we can do that, we may become like the immortals and "not show conventional signs of aging and (be) able to live beyond biological limitations" (Ni 1995, pp.3–4).

WHAT IS QIGONG?

Qigong ("chee gong") involves practices of unifying body, breath, and mind in order to attain and maintain ideal health. Throughout its development, qigong has been defined in various ways, but the core premise asserts that our internal energy can be strengthened with practice. "Qi" means "energy" and "gong" means "to cultivate with time and effort."

Practice implies dedication and perseverance over time to achieve a desired goal. *Body* refers to physical movements and anatomical structures. *Breath* regulation facilitates communication between the body and the mind. *Mind* refers to the power of intention and visualization. The focus on unification distinguishes qigong from other exercise systems. When we purposefully integrate specific body movements and coordinated breathing patterns with the mental intention to enhance and circulate our internal energy, we potentiate the power and function of those elements. As a result, we will enjoy the best possible state of health.

The many styles of qigong that developed through the centuries can be broadly categorized as either *external* with the qi directed outwardly, or *internal* with the qi guided inward. Between these two ultimate poles, further subsets of practice range from the very basic to the more advanced. For example, basic external forms stretch and strengthen the body, while advanced external practice could be projecting qi toward another person; basic internal forms harmonize breathing with tranquility of the mind, while advanced internal qigong could transform qi into Spirit. Most of the exercise sets practiced today blend both external and internal qigong styles, often with a bias toward one or the other.

Martial Qigong, an external form, builds strength from the inside out in order to develop an "iron shirt" for bodily protection and for projecting physical power. *External Qi Healing*, another external form, depends on the cultivation of the practitioner's internal qi in order to project this qi outward to another person. *Daoist Qigong*, in its advanced forms as an internal practice, promotes the dual cultivation of body and mind to awaken people's Spirits so they may realize their true humanity. The category of *Health Qigong* (*Jian Shen Gong*) combines internal and external qigong forms to varying degrees so that body, breath, and mind get nearly equal attention throughout a comprehensive practice. This qigong style provides an everyday exercise system that aims to strengthen the healing power of mind and body, thereby preventing illness and improving overall well-being. *Health Qigong* draws from many diverse energy cultivation techniques intended to nurture life and enhance health (Tianjun and Chen 2010, pp.5–8). While these four types of qigong exemplify stages of internal and external approaches, each remains more focused in one direction.

Qigong Through the Seasons, a type of *Health Qigong*, consists of external and internal exercises that tap into the healing energy within and all around you. The components of *Qigong Through the Seasons*—qigong, meditation, and diet—change when the four seasons change. The practice evolves throughout the year to maintain resonance with the seasons: winter practice with meditation, spring with body conditioning, summer with compassion, and autumn with boundaries. This seasonal variety keeps the practice interesting and refreshing, and very much in tune with the ongoing energy shifts in nature.

The qi from nature undergoes constant yin–yang transformations as the seasons change. You must synchronize your qi with nature's qi in order to be truly healthy. The powerful yin energy from earth and the limitless yang energy from heaven can be used to attain and maintain a state of optimum health. First you learn what to do, and then do what you learned.

QI

The vast concept of qi has no simple definition that can encompass its entire meaning. Chinese culture views it as the basic nature of everything from animals to plants, and mountains to planets. Qi is more than energy, more than matter, more than space. Qi embodies existence. Professor Ted Kaptchuk, an esteemed authority on Chinese medicine, explains it like this: "Everything in the universe, inorganic and organic is composed of and defined by its Qi.

Qi is not so much a force added to lifeless matter but the state of being of any phenomena" (Kaptchuk 2000, p.43). We can think of qi as being the intrinsic nature of a thing that gives it a form. For example, a tree roots to the earth for stability but reaches to the sun for energy—it is wide and deep at the bottom, but rises straight up to get close to the sun. The tree's innate qi gives it a narrow vertical form. The energy produced by photosynthesis, qi, keeps the tree alive. In its broadest sense, qi consists of both substance and power.

Qi has energetic properties recognized by modern science: electricity and magnetism in the body, gravity and radiation in the universe. Interesting research has been done on the electromagnetic forces of the human body. Becker and Sheldon (1985) cite studies done on the nature of acupuncture points and pathways. They found that the points had a greater electromagnetic charge than the surrounding skin. And when these points were mapped out on a significant number of subjects, they corresponded with the location of the acupuncture meridians. Matsumoto and Birch (1988) discuss how the electrical and magnetic fields of the body guide growth and healing from embryo to old age. They present fascinating research on human electromagnetic fields and their interactions with the environment. The universal forces of electricity, magnetism, gravity, solar radiation, and the subatomic nuclear forces are all part of the definition of qi.

In the practice of *Qigong Through the Seasons*, we think of qi as the vital energy within our bodies and minds, in food and herbs, and in all aspects of our immediate surroundings. Most of the qi that keeps us alive comes from what we eat and what we breathe. The nutrients and calories from food combine with the essential gases of the air to produce the nutritive energy that circulates through the meridian system to every cell of our bodies. In addition to the qi from food and air, we also absorb qi—consciously and unconsciously—from the environment. Some qigong exercises are primarily intended to bring energy from nature into our bodies; therefore we should practice in clean, fresh, natural surroundings.

YIN AND YANG

You are sitting on the side of a tall grassy hill in the late morning sun. You have hiked up from the lake below where you spent the night in a tent. The early morning air was very chilly down there beside the water, so you came up here for the warmth of the sun. As you sit and gaze out over the river valley, your cold hands and frosty face begin to thaw out in the heated air. It feels quite comfortable here as the sun rises further up the hill. Soon you feel pleasantly drowsy. You lie down on your back in the thick grass. Before long the sun feels hot on your face and you turn onto your side. As your mind slips into sleep the sun increasingly brightens the day. Then it reaches its zenith and begins to move to the other side of the hill. In time you wake up and feel a chill in the air. You sit up in shade. Here in the mountains the temperature changes rapidly with the ebb and flow of the sun's rays. Now you have become a little uncomfortable and begin to descend the hill in growing darkness. You have just experienced yin and yang.

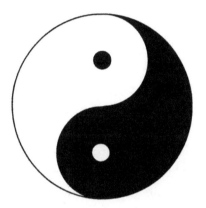

Figure 1.1: Yin–yang

Everything exists in a relationship to everything else. Nothing stays the same in nature. Change, metamorphosis, and recycling are constant aspects of life. The Chinese summarize this boundless perspective in the theory of yin and yang.

Yin and yang must, necessarily, contain within themselves the possibility of opposition and change...the (Chinese) character for yin originally meant the shady side of a slope. It is associated with such qualities as cold, rest, responsiveness, passivity, darkness, interiority, downwardness, inwardness, decrease, satiation, tranquility, and quiescence. The original meaning of yang was the sunny side of a slope. "The term implies brightness and is associated with qualities such as heat, stimulation, movement, activity, excitement, vigor, light, exteriority, upwardness, outwardness, and increase" (Kaptchuk 2000, p.8).

The palace of Chinese medicine stands on the foundation of yin–yang theory—a dialectical way of seeing the world and describing its contents. Yin and yang are not things; rather they serve as complementary and opposing labels that only exist in relation to each other. Take air temperature, for example. In general, winter is very cold, and summer is very hot. Spring and autumn temperatures lie somewhere between the extremes of winter and summer. The Daoist philosophers call winter the season of "Ultimate Yin"; spring the time of "Rising Yang," summer the season of "Supreme Yang"; and autumn the phase of "Descending Yin." This cyclical process of temperature fluctuation never remains still; it ceaselessly runs the circle of yin and yang transformation. Change, the crux of the theory, implies a constant revolution of yin qualities into yang qualities and vice versa. *Qigong Through the Seasons* emphasizes being attuned to these changes.

THE *DAN TIANS*

The Chinese term "*dan tian*" translates as "elixir field." Think of it as a place where energy (elixir) can be cultivated (like a farmer's field) with the practice of qigong. The *dan tians* function like deep quiet pools of water in the midst of a flowing river; they are reservoirs connected together by a current of qi. There are three major *dan tians* in the human body as shown in Figure 1.2.

The *lower dan tian* (LDT), located in the lower abdomen, receives the qi that the body produces from food and air. Like an alchemical stove, the LDT brews food essence and air essence into a wondrous elixir of pure energy. This vital qi reservoir must fill to capacity before that energy can be distributed though the meridian system. The *middle dan tian* (MDT), in the chest, receives the qi from the LDT and mixes it with blood from the Heart and Liver to give us the "HeartMind" (*xin*), a uniquely human quality created when emotions combine with intelligence. We connect with other people at the MDT. The *upper dan tian* (UDT), located in the head, combines the empathetic qi of the HeartMind with refined awareness and converts it into the human Spirit. This is the place where we make contact with all universal energies and experience spiritual awakening. The practice chapters later in this volume will present much more detailed information on the three *dan tians*.

The *dan tians* are located at regions of the body that have strong electromagnetic activity. The LDT relates anatomically to the small and large intestines. These organs are controlled by the enteric nervous system, which is sometimes referred to as the "second brain" because it can operate independently from the brain and spinal cord. The MDT harbors the Heart, and the UDT includes the eyes. The Heart and eyes generate the strongest electrical and magnetic fields in the entire body. Thousands of years ago, long before there was any such thing as modern scientific research, the sages and immortals of qigong developed such a refined and sensitive awareness of their bodies that they could detect, access, and enhance the functions of the three *dan tians*.

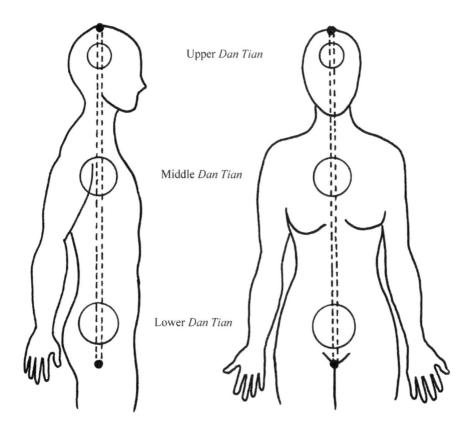

Upper *Dan Tian*

Middle *Dan Tian*

Lower *Dan Tian*

Figure 1.2: The three dan tians—LDT, MDT, UDT

TAIJI AXIS

The "*Taiji Axis*," as illustrated in Figure 1.3, is a flowing pathway for energy movement that runs vertically through the interior of the head and trunk, connecting the three *dan tians*. Acupuncture theory refers to this channel as the "Penetrating Meridian" (*Chong Mai*) and describes it as a conduit for the deepest energy circulation of the body and mind. The *Taiji Axis* forms an alignment between *huiyin* and *baihui*, which represent the lowest yin and highest yang areas respectively on the torso and head. Acting like magnetic poles, these two points serve as the prime movers of qi through this channel.

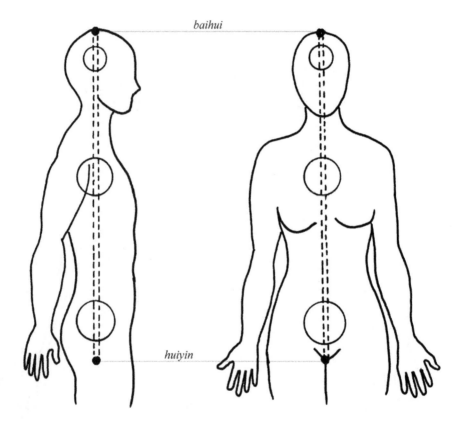

Figure 1.3: Taiji Axis—baihui, huiyin

In the higher levels of qigong practice, human beings are seen as the intermediary between earth and heaven ("heaven" meaning the forces generated from planets, stars, gravity, and radiation). In this context, *huiyin* represents earth and *baihui* symbolizes heaven. Some practices will bring Heaven Qi down through *baihui*, and Earth Qi up from *huiyin* to meet in the middle *dan tian* where these powers will enhance the awakening of the HeartMind for nurturing kindness and compassion.

The practice of *Qigong Through the Seasons* aims to open the *Taiji Axis* with qigong exercises and meditations. You will learn a range of effective and refined methods to energize this central channel so that your innate vitality is alive and well.

THREE TREASURES

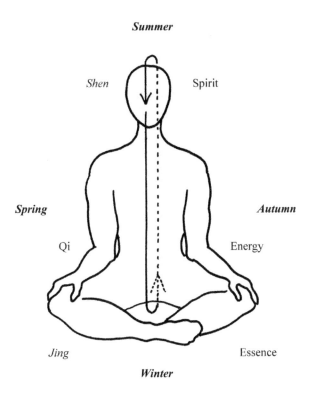

Figure 1.4: The Three Treasures/Seasons

Transform *Jing* into Qi,
Refine *Qi* into *Shen*,
Awaken *Shen* and
Return to the Void

(Cohen 1997, p.41)

This ancient statement from Daoist philosophy outlines the prime directive and ultimate purpose of a comprehensive Health Qigong practice. It begins with the fundamental substance of the body, develops the energy of body and mind, and eventually leads to a state of pure peace and fulfillment. *Jing*, *Qi*, and *Shen*, often translated as "essence," "energy" and "Spirit," are called the "Three Treasures" because they constitute the most precious aspects of our humanity. These are illustrated in Figure 1.4 on the previous page.

Jing means "essence." All organic life forms have essence. This essence contains the information and power that guides physical development. In the case of humans, we can think of *Jing* as our genetic code that determines how we grow and how we age. The majority comes from our parents, but some comes from foodstuff. The essence from our parents is called "prenatal *Jing*"; the essence from foods and herbs is "postnatal *Jing*." By and large, prenatal *Jing* accounts for most of the *Jing* in our bodies. Postnatal *Jing* from food does not guide our physical development, but nevertheless it enriches the parental essence and is vital to its manifestations. When we talk of *Jing* in the context of qigong practice we usually refer to prenatal *Jing*.

The form and function of our bodies expresses our essence. If we are born with a deficiency or abnormality of *Jing*, it can cause birth defects, atypical bone growth, dental problems, disorders of the central nervous system, and other conditions related to physical development. The important point to remember about prenatal *Jing* is that it comes in limited supply. We are born with all the *Jing* we will ever have. Every metabolic function that governs growth, sustenance, and repair consumes some of this essence. Stress and fear will definitely deplete essence. At the end of every day, we have less *Jing* than we did in the morning. And when we use up our supply of *Jing*, the body dies. The secret to longevity is to preserve the *Jing*; abundant good quality *Jing* makes the difference between senility and graceful aging. Longevity is part of human destiny; good *Jing* will increase the chances of enjoying it.

Prolonged illness or injury, excessive or inappropriate sex, poor diet, lack of sleep, and relentless stress all deplete our *Jing*. The ovaries, testes, bone marrow, and Kidneys store essence. Healthy Kidneys are essential for the preservation of *Jing*. Therefore, those qigong exercises that focus on the Kidneys establish an indispensable baseline of vibrant health. The primary focus of Winter Qigong is to protect and nourish the *Jing*.

Qi, as discussed above, means "vital energy." Most of our qi comes from food and air. The digestive system extracts the nutrients and energy from food; the Lungs take in oxygen and other vital gases from the air. Through a complex system of refinement and transportation, the elixirs of food and air combine in the LDT to create qi. Think of the LDT as a reservoir for holding Qi; when sufficient qi has filled that container, it will then flow out into the meridian system and circulate to every cell of the body. The important thing to remember is that the qi must first completely fill the LDT before it can be circulated through the channels. Therefore, almost all forms of qigong place great importance on cultivating the qi in the LDT as a basis for further practice. Qi is cultivated all the time in qigong, but it gets special attention in the spring and autumn seasons because the nature of qi rapidly changes from yin to yang and vice versa during these phases.

When we think of qi as energy, it suggests some type of force or power. This is a generally useful concept because qi is responsible for all movement and change in our bodies as well as in nature and the universe. But we should not limit our understanding of qi to only "energy." Some modern masters of qi theory advocate thinking of it in terms of information (Manaka, Itaya, and Birch 1995). Considering qi as a type of information helps us understand that qi can communicate through the body's meridian system, but also with other aspects of the environment. This broader definition means that qi involves a two-way street that can receive energetic information as well as project it. The ability to give and receive information is especially important at all levels of interpersonal communication, External Qi Healing, and when we are refining the qi in order to experience spiritual awakening.

Qi is depleted with excessive physical activity, discursive talking, and a poor diet. Intense exercise or hard work eventually exhausts the body; moderate exercise circulates and freshens the body's qi. Discursive speaking wastes physical and mental energy. Constant chatter and meaningless babble use too much Lung Qi and too little discernment. We should carefully choose what to say, and say it at the appropriate time. Conducting meaningful conversation will conserve your personal qi, and make you a more congenial person.

Shen, our "Spirit," distinguishes human life from animal life. This uniquely human Spirit combines our higher intelligence, mental intention, and emotional connections to form a recognizable personality. It becomes the self-awareness that seeks personal meaning and satisfaction as we go through life. When we nurture our *Shen* with qigong and meditation, we can develop an awareness of our destiny—our life path leading to a genuine feeling of fulfillment, self-worth, belonging, and contentment. *Shen* is like the light from a candle; it should glow brightly right up to the end.

Fear and anger dim the full light of *Shen*. Fear harms the Kidneys, and anger injures the Liver. Because the *Jing* and blood from these two organs merge in the UDT to nourish the *Shen*, anything that troubles the Kidney or Liver will diminish *Shen*'s full expression. The virtues of compassion and goodwill nurture the *Shen*; meditation and qigong practice cultivate these benevolent qualities.

The *Shen* also seeks a non-egocentric resonance with the world. In this case, the goal is to form a radiant empathic relationship with all sentient beings on earth and to express a deep stewardship for all organic and inorganic aspects of nature. A healthy human Spirit is at work when we become ardent conservationists, advocates for the unfortunate, landscape painters, or public servants working for the good of all citizens. Imagination, intuition, amazement, enchantment, creativity, morality, reverence, and purpose all come from a flowering Spirit. Remember, only when the *Shen* is awake can we become truly and completely human. Acts of kindness, benevolence, generosity, and compassion signal that the *Shen* has awakened to its true nature. Once that happens, the fully realized person—the sage—can return to the Void.

The "Void" does not refer to nihilistic meaninglessness. Rather, it describes an existential state of complete peace: a clear-minded view that everything is interconnected and functions as a unified expression of universal basic goodness. Daoists sometimes refer to "returning to the Void" as living in the womb of the Great Mother. All of the manifestations of spiritual awakening rise to a higher level. We attain a primordial state of pure mind—no prejudices or preconceptions, no craving or searching, no anger or fear. We attain a condition of selflessness, in which we are not separate from the present moment: we are fully alive, and our presence benefits the world.

The Three Treasures relate to the three *dan tians*—*Jing* resides in the lower, qi in the middle, and *Shen* in the upper. Think of the *Taiji Axis*. Because the human body has a vertical design, the alignment of the Three Treasures in their respective *dan tians* makes it possible for an upward and progressive refinement of these Treasures as we persevere in our qigong practice. In addition to being the abode of the Treasures, the three *dan tians* define regions on the *Taiji Axis* that house the deepest energy of earth, the fullest expression of humanity, and the highest inspiration of heaven.

Qigong practitioners can follow Daoism's prime directive in two ways: as a perpetual recycling of the Treasures where each can benefit the others, and as a single straight-line movement up the *Taiji Axis* to a final spiritual awakening. In the end, both paths happen together. Daily practice enriches the exchange of each Treasure as we go through life; *Jing* cultivation strengthens and protects the body, qi refinement energizes our social interactions, *Shen* awakening reveals our compassion and wisdom. This constant interplay of the Treasures makes life immensely satisfying and pleasurable. At the same time, over a long term of dedicated qigong practice, a gradual and unstoppable journey back to the Void also occurs. This dual process allows us to live each day with purpose and contentment, while eventually becoming a better person.

Keep in mind that *Jing*, *Qi*, and *Shen* interrelate and do not exist independently. They are not hard entities, but states of existence along the spectrum of yin and yang. Think of water. It comes in many forms: solid, liquid, vapor. Each existential form has its own characteristics: ice is extremely cold and dense, liquid moves freely and has weight, vapor rises upward and is warm. Ice exemplifies an extreme yin state of water, vapor is extreme yang, and liquid is middling. But they are all basically water. In a similar way, *Jing* and *Shen* represent different manifestations of qi.

Jing—a yin form of qi—relates to body structure and form. *Shen*—a yang form of qi—expands consciousness. Qi runs throughout the yin–yang continuum; it is the energy that brings about the appearance of yin or yang, and also stimulates their interacting transformations:

> The Dao gives birth to one, one gives birth to two,
> two gives birth to three, three gives birth to the ten thousand things.
>
> (Lao Tzu, Daodejing, Ch.42)

One = qi; two = yin/yang; three = *Jing, Qi, Shen*; ten thousand things = all objective and subjective phenomena in your life. The ultimate purpose of qigong is to attain good health. The prime directive provides a practical formula for living a full life. We are always living in the stream of these fundamental aspects of humanity, flowing toward the oceanic Void. We can use a qigong exercise to specifically cultivate one of the Three Treasures. As you have seen, in Figure 1.4 on page 35, each season of the year relates to *Jing*, qi, or *Shen*. Therefore, our *Qigong Through the Seasons* practice will focus on one of these treasures during each season.

CHAPTER 2

THE FIVE PHASES

INTRODUCTION

The Five Phases—*Wu Xing*—of Wood, Fire, Metal, Water, and Earth describe the interplay of forces that govern all changes in the universe. Every aspect of creation, destruction, and renewal on earth or in the heavens occurs within one of the Five Phases. When you understand interrelationships among the phases and how they affect your health, you can create a lifestyle that perfectly nourishes body, mind, and Spirit. The practice of *Yang Sheng*—Nurturing Life—includes qigong exercise, Daoist meditation, seasonal diet, and a deep connection with nature to help you achieve a life-nurturing state of equanimity and good health.

The Chinese phrase *Wu Xing* has been commonly translated in recent times as Five Elements. However, this translation is not entirely accurate. Wu means "five," and *xing* means "move, or walk," which implies a process. Most modern authorities (e.g., Beinfield 1991; Flaws 2010; Kaptchuk 2000; Needham 1978; Sivin 1987) render this term as "Five Phases" to more accurately express the inherent meaning of change, process, or cycle. Joseph Needham (1978) stated that *Wu Xing* refers more to five types of fundamental processes than to five types of fundamental matter. Paul Unschuld, the brilliant contemporary Sinologist, uses the term "agents" for *xing* because it conveys "the sense of forces that make certain things or processes happen" (Unschuld 2003, p.84). Whereas "element" has the sense of a structural substance, "phase" indicates moving from one thing to another. Some authors will use a combined translation, such as "Elemental Processes" or "Elemental Phases." But to be succinct and true to the original meaning, the term "Five Phases" will be used throughout this book.

The ancient Chinese Five Phases theory exemplifies the interdependence paradigm of modern physics: each thing in the world has a dependent connection to all things; nothing can exist without the supporting network of other objects and the universal patterns that connect them. Gregory Bateson, the great anthropologist and systems theorist, called these "metta-patterns" and said they are "primarily…a dance of interacting parts and only secondarily pegged down by…physical limits" (Bateson 1979, pp.12–14). Werner Heisenberg, a founder of Quantum Physics, echoed this ancient concept of interconnection when he explained that modern physics has divided the world, not into groups of objects, but into groups of connections that overlap or combine and thereby determine the composition of the whole. To make this idea even more comprehensive, Heisenberg went on to say, "The same organizing forces that have shaped nature in all her forms are also responsible for the structure of our minds" (Heisenberg 1971, p.101).

The Five Phases, always in perpetual motion, function as active cosmological energies. They form patterns of generation and control that create and maintain all organic life forms on earth. Furthermore, as these five powers recycle the seasons, control the tides, call up the sunrise, and keep our bodies alive, they are also responsible for the emotions, thoughts, and attitudes that make up our psyches. Each phase forms a network of correspondences made up of physical, mental, and spiritual traits that shape and direct the changes we go through from birth, growth, maturity, and decline to death. The system of correspondences comes from the indisputable influence of natural law on human health. It is absolutely imperative that we recognize and conform to the power of nature if we wish to avoid ill-health or disaster. Professor Paul Unschuld emphatically states that this is the basic message of *The Yellow Emperor's Classic of Medicine*, formally known as *Huang Di Nei Jing Su Wen*:

> …man has no way to manipulate the natural order…[it] has an unquestionable normative priority, and man must obey or perish. He cannot impose his will on nature. He is free to go with this order or to oppose it, but he cannot change it. (Unschuld 2003, p.124)

The annual seasonal cycle, well known to all earthly inhabitants, exemplifies the Five Phases in action. Everyone recognizes the changes among the four seasons. Some are as obvious as heat turning to cold, green leaves turning yellow, and long hours of daylight becoming shorter. But in the context of health, even more vital and subtle changes occur within our bodies and minds as the seasons progress. The Five Phases paradigm offers guidelines that help us live in harmony with these endless natural changes. Four of the phases— Wood, Fire, Metal, Water—have a correlated dominant season, internal organ system, emotional attribute, dietary preference, and other characteristics critical to healthy living at that time of year. The Earth Phase is special, as you will see. The basic premise of *Qigong Through the Seasons* recognizes that, because humans are part of nature, in order to be naturally healthy we must live in accord with energetic transformations that happen in the natural world. Staying tuned to the rhythms of life makes beautiful music.

Every student of Chinese medicine learns early on in their education this most fundamental tenet of good health as stated in the *Su Wen*: "For optimal health the qi and the blood must be abundant and freely circulating in body and mind." We need to have sufficient qi and blood, and it needs to flow without obstructions. Blood flows through the vascular system; qi flows through the meridian system. The meridian, or channel, system is one continuous circuit of energy flow, as Figure 2.1 shows. Often when people see a standard chart of the 14 major meridians, each with a specific label and numbering, they get the impression that each meridian begins at number one and ends with the last number.

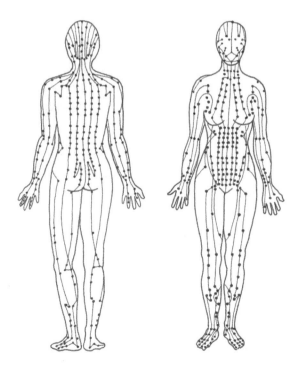

Figure 2.1: Meridian system

In fact, the numbers only indicate the location of those acupuncture points that are on the surface of the body and thus accessible to being stimulated with a needle or other tool. All meridians have deep pathways wherein they interconnect with those meridians that precede and follow in the order of the Qi Circulation Clock (see Chapter 5, page 74). The circulating energy should be like a great river rolling to the sea: active, powerful, and ever flowing.

While this incessant flow is continuing non-stop and without obstructions, there is also an accumulation of qi at certain areas of the body during each season. This collection of qi is like a deep pool at the bottom of the rushing river; the qi forms a reservoir that still has fresh energy flowing through it but with less speed and greater amassed energy. This seasonal circulation (Figure 2.2) correlates to the phases of Wood, Fire, Metal, and Water. We work with this energy when we practice *Qigong Through the Seasons*.

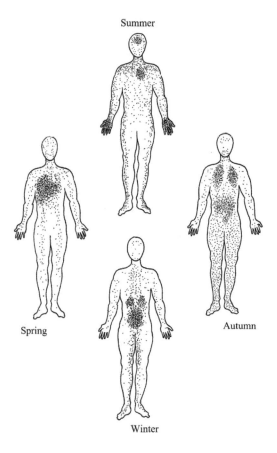

Figure 2.2: Seasonal circulation of qi

EARTH IS THE CENTER

Historically, the Earth Phase was graphically depicted as being the center, or pivot, around which the other four phases where circularly arranged. Several reasons for this are discussed below. However, today we commonly see the Five Phases illustrated with Earth on the circumference of a circle along with the other four phases (Figure 2.3).

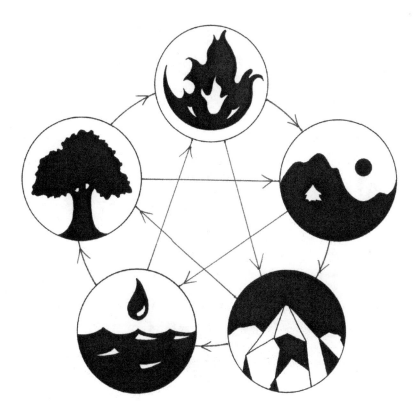

Figure 2.3: Five Phases

This ordering was made popular by The Five Element School of acupuncture founded by J. R. Worsley in the late twentieth century; they renamed the "phases" as "elements" and placed all five equidistant on a circle. While the Five Element acupuncture style is an elegant and often effective clinical system, it does not give Earth the special stature it has, and deserves, in the authoritative literature of Chinese medicine, such as *The Yellow Emperor's Classic of Medicine* (Ni 1995).

Earth is where we live. The comprehensive health care model presented in *Qigong Through the Seasons* teaches us how to live in harmony with the perennial changes happening on our home planet. We are creatures of the earth. Our lives are inexorably tied to its generative energy and to its countless energetic variables that influence our physical and mental health.

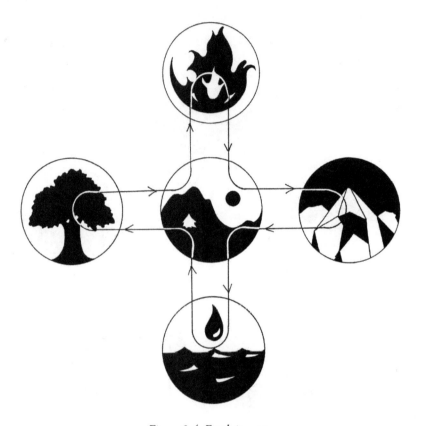

Figure 2.4: Earth in center

Earth constitutes the primary support of our existence; without it we could not be here. The textbooks of Chinese medicine emphasize the central importance of the Earth Phase: "Earth is the center of the five phases" (Flaws 2010, p.16). Because of its undeniable necessity, Earth—both planet and phase—should be located in the middle of the authentic Five Phases diagram (Figure 2.4) to indicate that it serves as an anchor as well as a transition among the other four phases. The ancient Daoist literature includes several examples where Earth resides in the middle of the arrangement.

The Wuji Diagram (Figure 2.5) historically validates the Earth-centric model. As a sophisticated representation of Daoist philosophy, this famous Sung dynasty rendering, when read from the top down, takes us through a numerical evolutionary process.

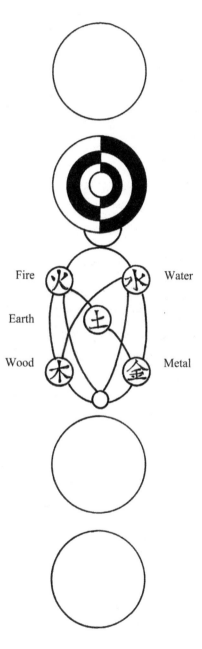

Figure 2.5: Wuji diagram

The empty circle at the top represents Wuji, "the Void," the Dao. The next circle down shows yin and yang, the interacting grand duality emanating from the Dao. Then the Five Phases are born from yin and yang with Earth in the center. The next circle down depicts the Male from Heaven and beneath that lays the Female from Earth. This dynamic transformative process, known as the Path of Generation, gives birth to all myriad things on earth and in heaven. When read from the bottom up, the Wuji Diagram (aka "*Taiji Tu*") maps out the Path of Return. The ultimate practice and goal of *Daoist Qigong* seeks to awaken the Spirit and "return to the Void." For a fascinating detailed description of this process, see Eva Wong's introduction to *Cultivating Stillness* (Wong 1992).

The Wuji Diagram has a curious arrangement in that Earth is placed in the center, which would obviously signify pivotal importance relative to the other peripheral four phases. And yet there is a connecting line running between Fire and Earth and between Metal and Earth, but no direction is indicated. In fact, the only sense of direction among the Five Phases is the vertical progression. And then there is that mysterious little circle at the bottom of the phases that has connecting lines from Wood, Fire, Metal and Water as seen in Figure 2.5. Other renderings of this diagram have that little circle connected only to Fire and Water (Wong 1992, p.xvi). This is a complex image whose multiple iterations may represent the changing philosophy of internal alchemy during the Tang and Sung dynasties. Several Daoist luminaries of that time—Chen Tuan, Wei Poyang, Lu Dongbin, Zhou Dunyi—may have contributed to the slight variations we have of the Wuji Diagram. Nevertheless, the fact remains that Earth is placed in the center of the other four phases in all variations. However nebulous these renderings may be, their predecessor in Five Phase philosophy was much more distinct.

The Yellow River Chart (*Hetu*) presents an even more ancient diagram of the Five Phases. We know it predates the Wuji Diagram, but its exact historical location remains unknown. The most accepted supposition holds that 4000–5000 years ago China's first emperor, Fu Xi, saw a dragon-horse (*longma*) emerge out of the Yellow River. As this semi-mythical animal shook itself dry, Fu Xi saw a pattern of black and white spots on its flank. The emperor discerned significance in the configuration of spots—he understood it to be a chart representing the transformation of yin–yang into the Five Phases. Fu Xi, the first of China's three legendary emperors of antiquity (the other successors are Shen Nong, the Divine Farmer, and Huang Di, the Yellow Emperor), had special perceptions and mystical knowledge of how the universe functioned. Based on his analysis of the *Hetu* he understood that Earth was the principle hub interlinking the other four phases and that if people would follow the diagram's numerical progression of change, they could predict and prepare for future environmental events such as floods, as well as use it as a form of medical prognoses. Ever since that primordial time, the Yellow River Chart (Figure 2.6) has been an invaluable source of knowledge to the philosophers and healers of China.

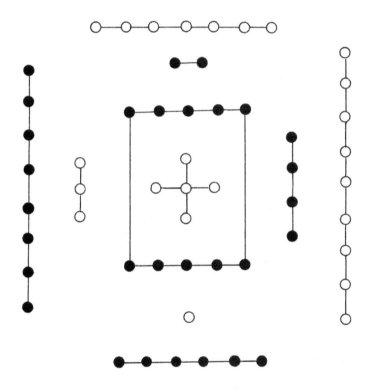

Figure 2.6: Yellow River Chart

As a mathematical model of the universe, this chart shows the complex permutations that occur through the interactions of yin and yang. The black even numbers represent yin and white odd numbers signify yang. There are five pairs of yin–yang numbers. You see that four pairs are arranged as a square and stand for Wood (left), Fire (top), Metal (right), and Water (bottom). The fifth pair of yin (10) and yang (5) numbers, signifying Earth, form a square within a square placed in the diagram's center. Each of the Five Phases has one smaller number and one larger number. The sum of all five small numbers is 15, and that of all five large numbers is 40; we now have two sets of numbers. The smaller set serves as the Engendering Code; the larger set defines the Completing Code. Daoist acupuncturists used these codes to determine point selection, and court officials used them to forecast how interactions and transformations of the Five Phases would affect virtually everything on earth: the weather, organ function, seasonal changes, fertility, even the destiny of the royal family. Modern Daoists still use them as venerable references for making treatment plans and prognostications, and performing geomancy (Liu 2008).

Another categorization of the phases especially useful for doing acupuncture and herbal treatments is built upon the idea that the expression of qi can be seen as increasing and decreasing yin or yang with, once again, Earth as the fulcrum. Qi constantly ebbs and flows through the world in cycles of creation and destruction so that an energetic equilibrium will prevail. "The Five Phases… articulate *ch'i* as greater and lesser *yin* (water and metal), greater and lesser *yang* (fire and wood), and a balanced center (earth)" (Oldstone-Moore 2003, p.64). We see that two of the phases are predominately yin, Water/Metal; and two are predominately yang, Fire/Wood. Yet within that overarching duality there are subdivisions, and even more subdivisions. Despite the seeming complexity, life exists in a narrow range of homeostasis maintained by Wood, Fire, Metal, and Water, beginning and ending in Earth. Good health depends on staying close to home. Each phase has a definite trajectory of yin or yang—increasing or decreasing—that would be unhealthy were it to progress unrestrained. But the eternal return to Earth mitigates excessiveness and restores an ideal harmony to our lives. Yin–yang theory may appear quite complicated, but its elegant and precise usefulness has enabled medical practitioners to form very specific treatment plans to effectively treat each person's unique syndrome of disharmony or disease.

For example, a healthy person will have Lesser Yin in the Metal Phase of autumn, which will inherently become Greater Yin during the Water Phase of winter. If the yin–yang progression continues naturally throughout the year, that person will have excellent health. A knowledgeable practitioner, after taking a detailed history and performing a competent examination, will diagnose the patient's condition as a permutation of excessive or deficient yin or yang; this determination will place them appropriately on the grand continuum of yin–yang interaction. The doctor will then recommend a treatment plan that brings the patient back into harmony with the cyclical changes.

The Wuji Diagram and the Yellow River Chart attempt to graphically explain how yin–yang dynamics produce the Five Phases and how these primordial powers engender all things in the universe. Because the ancient philosophers wanted to clearly conceptualize Earth's status relative to the other four, they placed it as the axis of the universal cycle. Likewise, *Qigong Through the Seasons* situates Earth as the pivot that each season-phase revolves around. In this scenario Earth does not have a related season because it functions as a grounding point to which the other phases return and pass through in their progressive transformations four times a year. Some scholar/practitioners consider the transition period of Earth to occur nine days before and nine days after each equinox and solstice (Wong 2000).

The relationship between the phases and diet plays an indispensable role in *Qigong Through the Seasons*. Each phase has foods and herbs that should be consumed during that time because they are beneficial to the organ and energetic systems associated with that phase. The Spleen and stomach organs are special in that they are associated with the Earth Phase and are largely responsible for metabolizing food, which is a predominant and constant concern of life. Although each seasonal chapter in this book has particular dietary recommendations, the guidelines presented in Chapter 4—spleen tonics, daily food, recipes—should be followed all year long. Earth is the eternal center of all changes.

UNDERSTAND THE PHASES FOR BETTER HEALTH

Healthy and unhealthy people all benefit from the practices in *Qigong Through the Seasons*. The anatomical structures, physiological functions, emotions, and virtues assigned to each phase are amenable to the rewards of doing qigong exercises and meditations, and using specific foods/herbs at the corresponding season.

Table 2.1 Five Phase Networks

	Wood	**Fire**	**Earth**	**Metal**	**Water**
Season	Spring	Summer	Transitions	Autumn	Winter
Yin and yang organs	Liver, Gallbladder	Heart, Small Intestine	Spleen, Stomach	Lung, Large Intestine	Kidney, Urinary bladder
Sense organ or orifice	Eyes, sight	Tongue, speech	Mouth, taste	Nose, smell	Ears, hearing
Flavor, color	Sour, green	Bitter, red	Sweet, yellow	Pungent, white	Salty, blue/black
Direction	East, upward	South, outward	Centre, stillness	West, downward	North, inward
Emotion, sound	Anger, shouting	Joy, laughing	Worry, sighing	Grief, weeping	Fear, groaning
Tissues and body parts	Muscles, tendons, fascia	Blood and blood vessels	Muscles, flesh/fat	Skin, nose	Bones, teeth, bone marrow
Spirit, virtue	*Hun*, kindness	*Shen*, compassion	*Yi*, harmony	*Po*, courage	*Zhi*, will/ wisdom

The organs, emotion, and bodily functions of the current seasonal network are most receptive to qigong practice during that time. Thus, as an example, a person with kidney disease should pay special attention to doing Winter Qigong because the Kidneys are open to stimulation at that time. On the other hand, each phase network has corresponding negative influences that can also affect our biology and psychology (e.g., Winter Qigong will also benefit a person who is fraught with worry and fear). Seasonal practice can both remedy an existing problem and prevent new problems from arising.

If the organs, systems, or thoughts belonging to each phase become too weak or too strong, they will show up as signs and symptoms of ill-health known as "patterns of disharmony" in Chinese medicine. If you know the harmonious appearance and function of these traits, you can recognize when things become imbalanced. *Qigong Through the Seasons* will show you how to recognize the most common disorders and what steps you must take to rebalance those discords.

When we live in harmony with the phases, we will be naturally healthy. Good health comes from taking in fresh environmental Qi and good food, dwelling in mental tranquillity, and doing meaningful movements, expressing appropriate emotions, and cultivating spiritual awareness. To do that we must be aware of how nature constantly reshapes our world throughout the year; when nature's essential energy changes, as it does with each season, it also changes accordingly within us. To live life to its fullest, we should follow the path of the Five Phases. If we consciously nurture the network of seasonal attributes, we will have a perfect practice for staying healthy throughout the year.

Each phase has a unique influence on every individual. Although we all, as members of the human family, have predictable and generalized responses to natural forces, each individual can also have a personal reaction to those forces. For example, someone who suffers from tension headaches, irritability, and muscle cramps will have a poignant relationship with the Wood Phase and the Liver organ because those are the symptoms of possible Liver dysfunctions. This person then should give special dedication to the practice of Spring Qigong. A person who has a history of bronchitis or asthma, and who is also unable to effectively set personal social boundaries, may have problems in the Lung Network; they should follow the training and emotional concerns of Autumn Qigong. You should practice throughout the year, but a particular season and phase may well have special significance for your current health status. If so, then practice during that season with more diligence and attention.

Everyone will gain unmistakable health benefits from following the program of *Qigong Through the Seasons*. If a person is "well balanced" and enjoys good health, they can maintain that state with this practice and even find higher levels of well-being. If an individual has specific health issues, they will certainly gain helpful information and particular techniques to improve their condition by practicing qigong, spending some time in meditation, and eating well. The practice of Nurturing Life, *Yang Sheng*, is for everyone who wants to be well in body, mind, and Spirit.

Chapter 3

Meditation

Mindfulness, Awareness,
Visualization, Awakening

The mind has, at least, two sides. It can create elegant mathematical order; it can compose stunning artwork; it can rectify inhumanity and rise above mere animal existence. But it can also, and often does, make us miserable. The tremendous capabilities of the mind can create both happiness and despair. At the core of our being exists an authentic, open, unbiased, loving, transcendent Spirit that strives for unity with people and place. But our essential nature often lies hidden beneath the travails and distractions of daily life, leaving us with a sense of lack, doubt, and insecurity. The ultimate awakening of the Spirit happens when we genuinely realize our interdependence with all things on earth and feel a wholehearted intimacy with the world. We have the ability to direct the mind toward positive states of health and well-being, but we often lose sight of our true nature because we become lost in the mind's wandering—its unfocused power scatters our energy, leading to distraction and confusion. As a result, our self-image becomes bewildered and complicated, which blinds us to our true nature and abandons us to suffering and ill-health. Happily, however, a remedy does exist: meditation can help us discover the peace and fulfillment that lies deep within our minds by teaching us how to stop restlessness, end discursive thinking, and drop negativity.

You will gather more information about specific types of meditation in each of the four seasonal practice chapters later in the book. For now, as you embark on a journey through your mind, you need to know that many meditations in the Daoist tradition have four aspects: mindfulness, awareness, visualization, and spiritual awakening. The first three aspects involve innate mental activities that can be used to train the mind—the fourth motivates training.

MINDFULNESS

Like a laser beam, mindfulness focuses on one and only one thing at a time. Being exclusive, the laser settles on a single object or activity and ignores everything else. The subject could be the breath cycle, a chant, a movement, or anywhere we want to place our full attention. When we immerse ourselves in mindfulness, we become completely absorbed in something without distractions. The process requires a certain willpower to develop concentration and mental stamina. The mindfulness that we cultivate in meditation becomes applicable to everything else we may do in our lives. As a technique for honing concentration and composure, practicing mindfulness helps control pervasive stress and daily diversions so that we become productive, attentive, and efficient. Mindfulness practice has become popular throughout society—in schools, offices, hospitals, and homes—because everyone benefits from having a calmly focused mind. And not just those mindful individuals: others around them benefit as well.

AWARENESS

Mental awareness observes our immediate world through sensory and cognitive perceptions. While mindfulness operates wholly in the present moment, meditative awareness has a sense of time to it—we were being mindful just a moment ago, but awareness notices that now we are not. Awareness notices when we lose concentration and will immediately bring our attention back to the object of mindfulness. It keeps us focused on a single task while at the same time it notices—but does not attach to—the streaming internal chatter, fantasies, and sensory details that occupy our thoughts. Awareness does not make judgments; it only observes how mindfulness ebbs and flows, but does not comment on it.

Mindfulness and awareness are the yin and yang aspects of meditation practice. Mindfulness remains profoundly still, exclusive, and internally directed. Awareness reaches out to be active, inclusive, and expansive. For example, when we concentrate on the breath cycle, mindfulness only feels the breath coming in and going out. Awareness knows we are breathing—but also feels the room temperature, hears the traffic outside, and notices when myriad thoughts have invaded our concentration and then gently brings our attention back to the breath. During a meditation session, the seamless interplay between mindfulness and awareness cultivates a conscious singularity that feels utterly peaceful, spacious, and clear.

VISUALIZATION

The use of intentional imagery expands the connection between body and brain, intensifies compassion, and develops spiritual awareness. Sport psychologists know that when we mentally imagine shooting a basketball it stimulates the same brain areas actually responsible for physically shooting the ball; this mental spark enhances the neural pathways for that action, which will make it familiar and more easily reproducible in the future. Research physiologists found that when long-term meditators practiced visualizing the dissemination of kindness and compassion to individuals or groups, the regions of the brain related to those emotions actually increased in size. The additional neurons of these regions raise the baseline for happiness in the meditator's mind, which imparts enduring tranquility, contentment, and benevolence.

Many Daoist meditation practices employ visualization to vitalize the body and expand the mind. The strategies often entail using specific imagery for improving qi and blood circulation through the meridian system, visualizing five healing colors for specific organs, or imagining a vivid journey to a sacred realm. There are also special meditations, which you will learn, that visualize an inner brilliant light rising up through the *Taiji Axis* and illuminating each energy center as it ascends to the upper *dan tian* where it kindles spiritual awakening, thus fulfilling the ultimate goal of qigong: the awakening of the Spirit and returning to the Void.

AWAKENING

Every person has a natural inclination to realize spiritual awakening. Consciously achieving an awakened state depends on cultivating the Three Treasures of humanity: essence, energy, and Spirit (see Chapter 1). An awakened Spirit truly understands interdependence and dwells in benevolence. As energetic beings we live in an ecosystem that begins deep inside the body, connects with the mind and emotions, interacts with natural and man-made phenomena, and extends into the boundless universe. We connect to everything that exists. Until we realize this universal bond—really feel it deep in the bones—we will continue living in alienation from our true self. When we have a profound comprehension and respect for our place in this ecology, and a genuine sense of generosity and good will toward all sentient beings, we will live in peace and harmony with the world. Spiritual awakening opens the door to selflessness and everlasting equanimity. Some people believe that spiritual awakening leads to divorcing oneself from society, but that does not hold true as long as you are living in your body on planet earth.

Once you experience enlightenment, you do not go away from the world; you remain fully invested in social engagements so that you can help others experience their true nature. Essentially, spiritual awakening can happen once or it can happen countless times, because the joy of living a fully realized life does not depend on time.

A well-functioning body and a tranquil mind are prerequisites for awakening the Spirit. To that end, we must diligently practice qigong, meditation, and healthy eating to set the stage for waking up. The more you practice meditation, the more skillfully you can create the process that leads to awakening. Just as importantly, moving qigong practice functions as a counterbalance to meditation—the Yang Qi that animates the Yin Qi of sitting.

Breath Counting—The foundation practice

Breathing functions as the most important thing we do from moment to moment; we cannot live without it. Because of this vital necessity, the technique of Breath Counting serves as the foundation for many meditation practices. Inhaling and exhaling connects our internal world with the external world, our body with our mind. The breath cycle exemplifies the perpetual link between yin and yang—we can't have one without the other; it provides a stable foundation for the mind and a gentle rhythm for the body when we are meditating. By counting each breath we are better able to clear our minds of distracting thoughts. All of us tend to carry on an incessant internal dialogue of always talking to ourselves, which often carries a tinge of negativity. The rambling chatter creates a pervasive tension in the mind and thus in the body. Breath Counting dampens the chatter so that our mind can be clear, open, and receptive. It is a simple practice, but far from easy.

Begin by sitting upright on a cushion or chair. Hold your spine comfortably erect with hands resting on thighs with palms down, or in your lap with palms up and one hand on top of the other. If you sit on a meditation cushion (zafu), your knees should be bent and legs crossed in one of the following positions: both feet on the floor one in front of the other (natural lotus position), or one foot resting on the lower leg of the other (half lotus), or both feet resting on the lower part of the opposite leg (full lotus). If sitting on a chair, your feet should be flat on the floor; the chair seat should also be flat to facilitate uprightness. You may also choose to sit on a specially designed bench (seiza) where the lower legs tuck beneath the seat. A timer can be helpful to set an allotted period to practice: 10, 20, 30 or more minutes are good options.

Relax, and just become aware of your breath coming in and going out. Don't try to control the cycles, just watch them. The breath cycle has four stages: inhalation, pause, exhalation, and pause. Again, put your attention on the breath cycles for a minute or two; become aware of the four parts of breathing. Notice how the pause after exhalation extends out longer than the pause after inhalation. Daoists call that lingering pause after exhaling "a moment of immortality."

Now, begin to silently count your exhalations from one to ten. Notice what happens. Many thoughts will flicker through your mind. The goal is to not become attached to those thoughts; don't dwell on them. You simply keep letting go of the thoughts and constantly bringing your mind back to the count. If you forget the count, just go back to one. Relax. Almost everyone will lose track of the count at times because a thought carried their mind away. It commonly happens. The most important issue is that you do not get caught up in self-criticism—no judgments—just come back to the breath. If you do reach the count of ten, return to one and continue counting the exhalations up to ten again, and again. Eventually you will become peaceful and undisturbed by the thoughts that move through your mind like clouds across the sky. Then, after the chosen time has expired, let go of counting the breath and simply rest in tranquility. Let that moment of immortality linger a little longer.

You can use Breath Counting as a stand-alone meditation, or you can use it as an adjunct to a qigong and/or seasonal meditation session. Mindfulness and awareness—

the cornerstones of meditation—will carry your mind along the breath toward equanimity and good health. However you use it, the breath cycle will always be available to assist in the discovery of your true nature.

CHAPTER 4

FOOD, HERBS, AND THE FIVE PHASES DIET

Everyone wants to be healthy so they can enjoy a long and happy life. This universal desire has motivated the medical use of food and herbs throughout human history. Over the last 3000 years, the Chinese have researched and developed a magnificent herbal medicine and food therapy system that fosters optimal health and longevity. Chinese culinary philosophy has an indistinct boundary between food for eating and food for healing. In some respects, Chinese cuisine's distinctive appeal comes from using herbs for both flavor and health.

Often times, the difference between a condiment and a medicine only differs by degree. Take ginger, for example: as a common ingredient in many recipes it imparts a pungent, warming taste much enjoyed by countless diners around the world. At therapeutic dosages, ginger can be used to dispel upper body congestion, phlegm, and viral invasions; it can also help alleviate menstrual cramps, motion sickness, and indigestion. Consequently, ginger can be used as a spice and/or a remedy. In Chinese cooking, plants may be used for flavoring or for healing; the use depends on the intention. Of course every culture has, to some extent, used food for healing throughout its history, but the Chinese have attained unmatched accomplishments in both sublimely delicious cuisine and unparalleled medical herbalism. Nevertheless, caution is warranted because some herbs can involve risks when used at medicinal dosages. Only use particular substances for specific remedial or therapeutic purposes in consultation with a licensed health care practitioner.

Humans reflect the universe. All cosmic energies are mirrored in us so that as heaven and earth energy circulates in seasonal planetary cycles, it also moves in natural patterns within us. In spring the energy comes up through the solar plexus; in summer the energy moves to the head and the extremities; in autumn the energy retreats toward the trunk; and in winter the energy moves down and inward to the body's core. Eating specific foods at each season can influence how the internal qi circulates. A plant's growing shape, what herbalists call the "doctrine of signatures," supports this movement within us: eat upward sprouting food in spring, flowers and leaves that grow outward in summer, downward growing vegetables for autumn, densely concentrated grains, seeds, and nuts in winter. Naturally, we prefer to eat fruits and vegetables as they ripen. They taste so good because they contain the plants' full growth and ultimate vitality, and we should eat them before that energy wanes. *Qigong Through the Seasons* encourages wise use of seasonal specific foods and herbal tonics to maintain good health and vitality. The dietary information that follows will generally promote healthy digestion. While not intended to prevent or cure any specific disease, it will improve your functional nutrition so that you get the most from what you eat.

SEASONAL DIET

You learned in Chapter 2 that the Five Phase model assigns environmental, physical, mental, and spiritual correlations to each phase in the yearly cycle. The environmental and physical categories include the seasons, organs, directions, and flavors. These are the tangible aspects of each phase—structure, movement, and sensation—that comprise the essence of the body's reality, the ground upon which mind and Spirit stand.

> Wood—spring—Liver—upward—sour.
>
> Fire—summer—Heart—outward—bitter.
>
> Earth—transition—Spleen—central—sweet.
>
> Metal—autumn—Lungs—downward—pungent.
>
> Water—winter—Kidneys—inward—salty.

The Five Phases diet recommends using foods and herbs that do two things: 1) nourish a specific organ with tonic herbs and 2) harmonize the body's energy with the season's energy by eating appropriate food. For example, foods and herbs can influence three important aspects of the Wood Phase: the Liver, Rising Qi, and the sour flavor. Specific tonic herbs provide nourishment to the Liver, and the sour flavor cleanses it of metabolic debris; upward-growing vegetables carry the Rising Yang Qi of spring and when eaten can augment our own Rising Qi. So if you want a healthy Liver, your spring diet will include sour foods such as yogurt, citrus fruits, and rhubarb; herbal tonics made from bupleurum, dandelion, and milk thistle; and your meals will include upward-growing vegetables such as asparagus and romaine lettuce. This book presents detailed guidelines for each season in its respective chapter.

Eating locally grown food provides many benefits: fresh food tastes great; it has micronutrients from local soil; it contains environmental qi from the landscape; and local plants breathe the same air that you do. These subtle, but vital, interactions between food, you, and the environment provide unique energies that potentiate the power in the plants. However, non-native foods and herbs may also play an important part in a healthy seasonal diet.

Insatiable curiosity compelled ancient people from diverse cultures to travel the world by land and sea searching for foods and medicines that were different, and perhaps more useful, than what was found in their native lands. They crisscrossed the continents of Asia, Africa, Australia, Europe, and the Americas to discover and collect new plants. The period from the eleventh to the fifteenth centuries was an extraordinary time of cultural exchange around the globe. These voyagers returned home with strange, exciting plants and got busy conducting investigations into their health-promoting properties. They discovered ways to extract the medicinal essence and preserve it for future use; and they found ways to successfully grow many of these plants in their own environment. Eventually, these endeavors enabled people to grow and use assorted foods and medicinal herbs during any season or weather.

Early healers could employ this rich diversity in their quest to improve individual and community welfare. Today, medicinal herbs and seasonal guidelines continue to have a place at the table of healthy eating. The Five Phase diet strongly recommends using both fresh and preserved plants for their specific nutritional, medicinal, or energetic benefits at each season. The guidelines for each seasonal phase are detailed in the practice section of *Qigong Through the Seasons*. Following them means that the seasonal dietary ingredients will change over the year.

However, your constant need for a properly functioning digestive system never changes; it is the engine driving the conversion of food to qi.

DAILY DIETARY GUIDELINES

Your Spleen and stomach, the principle organs of the Earth Phase, are responsible for digesting and assimilating everything you eat. Optimal digestion depends on the Spleen being healthy and fully functional. As two scholars have succinctly stated, "In Chinese medicine, healthy digestion is synonymous with a happy *Spleen*" (Beinfield and Korngold 1991, p.327). The Spleen and stomach will be "unhappy" if they are congested with mucus and phlegm, if food and drink are too cold, and if you are mentally mired in worry and rumination. To enjoy good health, we must extract nourishment from food and drink at each meal, and soon thereafter we must eliminate the by-products. As you can see, the Earth Phase plays an essential role, every day, in your well-being.

The Spleen and stomach transform what we eat into usable and unusable products. The stomach first soaks the food with digestive enzymes and then uses its powerful muscles to break down the contents into manageable particles; secondly, the stomach transports the macerated food through the intestines for further processing. The Spleen governs the entire digestive process, including those functions of the stomach, Liver, gallbladder, and pancreas that convert food into essential energy and nutrients. The medical classics identify this Earth organ as the essential core of digestion; "The spleen is the root of the central Qi" (Flaws 1994, p.59). The central qi travels through the *Taiji Axis*; therefore, to ensure healthy digestion and abundant energy throughout the three *dan tians*, we must keep the Spleen happy. The following information highlights safe and effective herbal tonics and foods that can boost your health status by improving gastrointestinal function.

SPLEEN TONICS

The "Four Gentlemen Decoction" (*Si Jun Zi Tang*)—a very famous herbal formula for Spleen Qi Deficiency—contains ginseng, atractylodes, licorice, and poria. These "four gentlemen" from the herbal kingdom, when combined in equal parts, can gently and effectively improve digestion and elimination. As always, a qualified practitioner should be consulted before taking these or any other medicinal herbs. The standard ingredients include the following popular tonic herbs:

- *Ginseng (ren shen)*—stimulates food metabolism, improves appetite and transit time in the gut, strengthens overall energy, and protects the Spleen's Yin Qi.

- *Atractylodes (bai zhu)*—increases general Spleen Qi, rectifies loose bowels, relieves bloating, and strengthens the Yang Qi.

- *Poria (fu ling)*—eliminates excessive dampness in the spleen and gas in the gut, strengthens the Yang Qi.

- *Licorice (gan cao)*—harmonizes the relationships among the other herbs for smooth and gentle action.

The sweet and bitter herbs in this tonic will effectively and gently relieve the following Spleen Qi Deficiency symptoms: fullness and bloating in the abdomen or chest, discomfort in the stomach, belching, flatulence, general lassitude, poor appetite, and loose stools. These herbs are usually taken in capsule form. Dosage should follow label directions, starting with lowest dose first. A good herbalist can modify the proportions, or add other spleen tonics, for a more specific therapeutic effect.

UNREFINED COMPLEX CARBOHYDRATES

Carbohydrates are the main food source for qi production. Ideally, we want an adequate and steady energy flow to muscles, organs, nerves, and the brain as a stable and continuous supply maintains healthy tissue function throughout the body. We do not want sharp and sudden energy spikes followed by steep declines as dramatic fluctuations can lead to hypoglycemia and possibly diabetes. The best energy comes from complex carbohydrates—starches—such as oats, rice, barley, corn, wheat, potatoes, legumes, fruits and vegetables. Simple carbohydrates—sugars—include sucrose, glucose, fructose, honey, lactose, dextrose, and maltose, which are rapidly absorbed and, if not immediately used for energy, quickly converted to fat. Unrefined complex carbohydrates are better than the processed variety because they retain more healthy fiber, have more nutrients, and slowly release their energy. The concept is not complicated: steel-cut oats are better for you than rolled oats; wholegrain brown rice is healthier than white rice.

Oats and rice are among the most widely eaten grains on the entire planet: oats in the northern hemisphere and rice for the southern portion of the globe. These hypoallergenic, complex carbohydrates have nurtured earth's people for ages. Their benefits to humanity cannot be overstated. Undeniably, modern genetic engineering has altered many cereal plants, especially wheat. We are seeing more problems with gluten intolerance every year, but this is primarily a concern with wheat because it is the most widely consumed grain on this planet and has had the greatest amount of genetic manipulation. Unadulterated oats do not contain gluten, but they can be tainted by wheat grown nearby; rice, too, has no gluten and does not grow in the same environment as wheat. For these reasons, pure oats and rice are well digested by most people.

Oats offer a perfect way to start the day. They contain seven B vitamins, Vitamin E, nine minerals, and gamma linoleic acid (GLA)—an essential fatty acid. Oats have, ounce for ounce, twice the protein found in wheat or corn, and they are naturally gluten free. Oats are exceptionally nutritious because they have beta-glucan and avenanthramides. Beta-glucan, a special soluble fiber that gives oatmeal its creamy texture, can significantly lower cholesterol levels in the blood; oats contain more beta-glucan than any other grain. Avenanthramides, a unique antioxidant compound, prevents cholesterol molecules from attaching to blood vessel walls—thus lowering the chances for developing atherosclerosis and other circulatory problems.

Because they contain these special nutrients, oats have a well-deserved reputation for protecting the cardiovascular system. Steel-cut oats provide more heath benefits than rolled or "quick" oats since they have more fiber and a lower glycemic index that keeps blood glucose at a healthy level. Steel-cut oats take longer to cook than the more processed type, but the gain in nutritional value is well worth the wait. The following preparation method works very well:

---------------- Cooked Oats ----------------

(Makes 3½ cups)

Boil water in the bottom pan of a double boiler. Place ⅔ cup of steel-cut oats in the top pan. Rinse and drain with fresh water. Add two cups water to oats (more or less for desired thickness).

Place the pan of oats on top of the pan of boiling water. Reduce heat and simmer for 45 minutes.

Leftovers keep well in the refrigerator for up to three days. Simply reheat in the microwave oven or on the stovetop. Add nuts, fruit and/or a little sweetener.

CONGEE

Congee, a rice gruel or porridge commonly found in Asian diets, has unlimited uses as an easy-to-prepare and very healthy meal. This dish even becomes a medicinal tonic if herbs are included in the recipe. Simple to make and incredibly adaptable, congee can include various herbs, vegetables, meats, and flavorings. Cooking is quite easy: simmer one part rice in five-to-six parts water until thoroughly cooked, usually in one to two hours. Adjust the water amount to make a thinner or thicker porridge.

The basic recipe usually includes some vegetables. Add chopped celery, spinach, and bean sprouts as cooking progresses. For an especially warming congee, add diced fresh ginger at the start, or add lightly stir-fried vegetables just before serving. Cucumber and water chestnuts promote internal cooling so they can have a nice refreshing effect in hot weather. Gentle medicinal herbs can be added in small amounts. Astragalus, *Huang Qi*, is a favorite winter congee ingredient due to its warming and immune supporting effects. Remember to always consult a qualified practitioner if you want to add herbs for a particular remedial effect.

When eaten for breakfast, congee recipes should be kept rather modest— perhaps just a little celery or ginger added with the rice. But adding more substantial ingredients, such as thinly sliced meat or root vegetables, also works well for lunches and dinners. Simplicity and flexibility make congee an attractive choice for keeping meals nutritious and appealing.

BRASSICA VEGETABLES

If you truly want to have a healthy diet, you will definitely include vegetables from the *Brassica* family as these superfoods are exceptionally valuable for reducing inflammation and eliminating toxins in the body. Researchers no longer use the older term "cruciferous" for these plants because that name referred to the cross-shaped leaves of some members in this group, but not all *Brassica* vegetables have leaves shaped like a crucifix. Therefore, "*Brassica*" is the preferred term because it identifies this group of plants by their genus name. These vegetables are packed with powerhouse nutrients shown to have anti-cancer, and what some call anti-aging, benefits. The most commonly consumed plants in this group include arugula, bok choy, broccoli, Brussels sprouts, cabbage, cauliflower, kale, turnip, and radish.

These deep green, pungent vegetables are packed with the conventional vitamins—A, B, C, folic acid—plus healthy doses of calcium, iron, sulfur, and zinc. The astonishing Vitamin K, which has clearly shown its ability to reduce chronic inflammation that can lead to cancer and other chronic conditions, is found in most *Brassica* food but is especially abundant in kale. Broccoli has more Vitamin C than citrus fruit; kale has more Vitamin A than carrots; cabbage has aromatic sulfur that can combat inflammation and assist in calcium absorption.

These plants have a bitter taste, and that is a good thing because the bitterness comes from the health-enhancing phytonutrients contained within them. The glucosinolates, dithiolthiones, and indoles are especially impressive in their cancer prevention capabilities. The bitter flavor corresponds to the summer Fire Phase and to the Heart. Bitterness will cool heat in the blood and clear stagnation in the circulatory system. Bitter foods can also resolve damp conditions that cause excessive mucus, edema and some skin eruptions. Many Westerners shun bitter food for one reason or another; unfortunately, they miss out on many benefits provided by these immune-system-enhancing foods.

Without a doubt, you should eat *Brassica* vegetables often and in generous portions. Because these foods provide complex carbohydrates (the same as oats and rice), the body can slowly use their energy over a sustained time; their high fiber keeps the digestive system clean and smooth; and their nutrients are steadily absorbed for long-term use. They can be eaten raw or cooked. To receive their full enzymatic and vitamin complements, you must eat these plants within 48 hours of their being harvested; otherwise, their vitamin content rapidly declines. Lightly steaming *Brassica* foods depletes some metabolic enzymes, but the benefits gained from pre-digestion, warm temperature, and better nutrient availability—indoles, for example, are only formed when the plant is cooked— outweigh the minor losses.

RAW VS. COOKED

The temperature inside the stomach is about 100°F (37.7°C). At that warmth, enzymes and stomach acids can efficiently break down the contents. If the ingredients consumed have temperatures much less than 100°F, the stomach will have to put energy into heating them—energy that should be used for digesting food. Lightly frying, steaming, or sautéing enhances digestion. Cooked food also releases aromas and flavors, which tickles the appetite and awakens the senses with pleasant anticipation. Time-honored cooking methods such as stir-frying and light sautéing present food at its best. Refrigerated food generally should be brought to at least room temperature before eating. Frozen foods must be reserved for occasional treats as they drastically reduce stomach temperature; there should be at least ten minutes between the end of a meal and serving a frozen dessert.

Liquids, too, should be consumed at nearly the same temperature as the stomach. When boiling water is poured into a cup at room temperature, it takes about 15 minutes to cool down to 100°F. This feels tepid; many prefer their warm beverages to be about 110–115°F (43.3–46.1°C). Liquids above 120°F (48.8°C) will cause most people to perspire. Tea, nature's healthiest drink, makes a wonderfully warm accompaniment for many meals; especially for breakfast and lunch since it contains a little caffeine. Tea comes in three major styles—green, oolong, and black—that allow for interesting tea and food combinations. If liquids are not warm, they should be cool and thirst quenching, but not too cold, and rarely iced. Simply taking in warm food and drink will help the stomach efficiently and comfortably convert food to qi.

The great debate regarding the relative superiority of raw or cooked food has no single simple answer. The choice depends on the food and the person's needs. Overcooking, by definition, is not good. Briefly cooking most foods, or at least warming them up to room temperature, will increase the availability and assimilation of their nutrients; what little enzymes or other constituents may be lost is not significant relative to the gain in nutrition and energy. In general, you should eat complex carbohydrates such as vegetables and grains, cooked; simple carbohydrates, such as fruits, may be eaten raw. Of course, there are always exceptions. Realistically, sometimes cold, uncooked food will be appropriate, and raw salads seem like the right thing to eat. And, occasionally, they are. The final decision depends on what makes a person feel good. Eating should be a pleasant experience. If you are bloated, agitated, or have any other undesirable feelings during or after a meal, you should look to the type of food you just ate and how it was prepared.

These days, making dietary decisions can be quite difficult due to the unrelenting promotion of multifarious meal plans that come our way in media and advertising. Some regimens are so complicated they discourage, some so restrictive as to be joyless, and some so time consuming they are unworkable. Again, no one diet will suit everyone optimally. But generally the diet that is straightforward, adaptable, and true to whole foods will offer a sound choice. A naturally healthy diet centers on local foods as they grow and mature, as well as those herbs and foods that can synchronize our personal energy with nature's great encompassing seasonal energy.

The Five Phases diet suggests that everyday meals should include gentle tonic herbs, oats, rice, and *Brassica* vegetables in various combinations. Additionally, you should add certain herbs and food groups to your diet at particular times. You can find more detailed information in the specific chapters on seasonal practice. Keep the primary diet simple: choose many foods with different colors, briefly cook them, and have tea with some meals.

You should enjoy a meal calmly and completely. Obsessing over "good" or "bad" foods has little practical value. Of course, a genuine food allergy should be taken seriously and warrants professional advice, but—for most people—a well-rounded diet incorporating the food suggestions above will serve them well. As your qigong and meditation practice advances, your awareness becomes more attuned to how food reacts in your body: you will know which foods are good for you—they feel right—and which should be avoided. This subtle inner awareness is a key component of healthy eating; the best way to develop it is with dedicated internal qigong practice. Always remember that digestion functions best with warm, aromatic, and tasty food. Eating should be a time when you relax and enjoy the miraculous transformation of food into qi.

CHAPTER 5

CHRONOBIOLOGY

INTRODUCTION

Put your fingers over the pulse at your wrist. Press lightly. Thump, thump, thump. You are feeling time. The rhythm of the pulse signals life in the body. No beat, no time, no life. Time equals movement; one moment becomes the next. Life takes place over time: blood flowing through the vessels, the lungs breathing in and out, and the seasons changing one to the next.

Chronobiology is the study of how time affects living organisms. Cycles and transformations control the existence and demise of all life forms. A red blood cell lives for 120 days; a white blood cell lasts for more than a year. Cells in the colon die after four days; sperm cells wear out after only three. Each type of cell is then reborn for another time. The body has a tempo within itself, but at the same time it is influenced by terrestrial and celestial rhythms. There are many cycles, with differing rhythms, that powerfully affect human health.

The circadian rhythm (*circa*: about; *diem*: a day) is what we call the 24 hours in the day/night cycle. Sleep is the most important human event that happens in the circadian cycle. Disruptions in the sleep–wake cycle can affect the whole person, causing anything from mild irritability, to distressing jet lag, to potentially fatal depression. Research has identified other definite 24-hour cycles in brain wave activity, immune cell production, and hormone levels. For example, the intimate relationship between peak levels of male testosterone and female ovulation results in the ideal time for getting pregnant. Testosterone reaches its peak between 4:00 am and 8:00 am. High progesterone levels and ovulation occur between midnight and 2:00 am. Together, these events make the chances for conception to be greatest between 6:00 and 8:00 am (Foster and Kreitzman 2004).

The Qi Circulation Clock represents a very important circadian cycle. This concept goes back to early Daoist philosophy. The Clock illustrates how energy flows through the body's 12 major meridians. Each meridian and its corresponding organ have a two-hour period when the qi flow reaches its maximum and an opposing two-hour period when it is minimum. The times when the meridians are replete with qi are:

11:00 pm–1:00 am: Gallbladder

1:00 am–3:00 am: Liver

3:00 am–5:00 am: Lung

5:00 am–7:00 am: Large Intestine

7:00 am–9:00 am: Stomach

9:00 am–11:00 am: Spleen

11:00 am–1:00 pm: Heart

1:00 pm–3:00 pm: Small Intestine

3:00 pm–5:00 pm: Urinary Bladder

5:00 pm–7:00 pm: Kidney

7:00 pm–9:00 pm: Pericardium

9:00 pm–11:00 pm: Triple Heater

Qi volume in a meridian bottoms out 12 hours after the peak. Qi normally ebbs and flows between fullness and emptiness. Symptoms of excess qi become more intense at times of peak qi volume, while symptoms of deficiency get worse in the valley. For instance, heart attacks most commonly happen around noon, while heart failure usually occurs around midnight. In the case of asthma and obstructive lung disease, characterized by excessive chest tension and fullness, most attacks occur very early in the morning.

Qigong practice and acupuncture treatments can be exceptionally helpful in treating imbalances of qi circulation. Some astute health care practitioners will pay close attention to the time when their patient's symptoms occur and may use that to diagnosis the problem. Treatments may be performed at the high or low points of qi circulation depending on the condition. Timing is very critical in classical Daoist acupuncture practice. Dr. Liu Zheng-Cai places supreme importance on circadian qi circulation when formulating a treatment strategy.

> When using Daoist methods of point selection, time is the key factor. In other words, which acupoint, or group of points, is chosen is decided by time regardless of the nature of the patient's condition or the actions of the points. (Liu 2008, p.125)

An ultradian rhythm is shorter than a day (i.e., it has a frequency that occurs more often than a circadian rhythm). The heart beats about 70 times a minute; a healthy breath cycle is about eight seconds for most people. At night, the four stages of normal sleep occur in 90-minute cycles. These vital cycles keep us functioning from moment to moment. If we didn't have ultradian rhythms we couldn't have a circadian rhythm.

And then there are the infradian rhythms, which have periods that are longer than a day and happen more often than once a year. The two most well-known infradian rhythms—the menstrual cycle and the lunar cycle—are about 29.5 days each. This synchronization between a biological rhythm and a celestial event beautifully illustrates how closely we are connected to nature. Rhythms that are influenced by the phases of the moon are called circalunal. These cycles impact countless events on our planet: the oceanic tides, the procreative activities of innumerable animal and plant species, and the variations in the human body's electromagnetic field, to name a few.

Finally, there are the circannual cycles that last a year. Human society has been aware of these annual rhythms in nature for millennia; it has, in fact, been dependent on understanding some of them—migration, hibernation, plant flowering, and animal reproduction—for its survival. Because each season has unique characteristics that are vital to our lives, the unending change through the four seasons of spring, summer, autumn, and winter is by far the most important circannual cycle for human existence

Seasons are not only about the weather. While all environmental events do have an impact on our lives, it is the subtle but powerful internal forces that create our health. The cyclical manifestation of these forces in our bodies—*Qi*, *Jing*, and *Shen*—is definitely linked to the ever-changing nature of the seasons.

Chronobiology has always been integral to human health care. Every culture, to some degree, has recognized the relationship between time and biological events. The Chinese have one of the oldest civilizations on earth and have studied astronomy for over 4000 years. They developed elegant theories regarding the effect of celestial–terrestrial interactions on human society. They came to understand that if people knew the impact of seasonal changes on themselves, and if they lived in accord with the conversion of one season to the next, they would experience good health, peaceful prosperity, and social solidarity. This is summed up in *The Yellow Emperor's Classic of Medicine*: "He who would nourish life surely follows the changes of the four seasons, adapts to cold and heat, harmonizes joy and anger, and dwells in calm" (cited in Flaws 1994, p.14).

The science that studies events in time, *chronology*, was highly developed by the ancient Chinese as shown in the lunisolar calendar where they calculated time according to both the moon phases and the "solar terms." In this calendar, a year usually begins on the second dark/new moon after the Winter Solstice. Each subsequent new moon begins another month. The lunisolar calendar also has solar terms, each about 15 days that are arranged around the Summer and Winter Solstices, and the vernal and autumnal equinoxes. It gets even more elaborate: four solar terms equal 60 days. A 60-day period is called a "step." Six steps equal one year. Then there are 60-year cycles, which form the basis of Chinese astrology. This system's complexity can be distilled into the premise that time exists in repetitive cycles that can be observed and calculated. And since our lives are inextricably tied to time, we cannot live outside these cycles; the four seasons are the most important cycle that influences the state of human health and society.

When does a season begin? Is the Summer Solstice actually the beginning of summer? Or is it the middle of summer as depicted in Shakespeare's *A Midsummer Night's Dream*? Is the Winter Solstice, which has the longest night of the year in the northern hemisphere, the beginning of winter or does it mark the mid-point of the season because daylight hours are increasing?

Seasons are generated by the amount of solar radiation hitting the earth's surface. Sunlight primarily determines ambient air temperature. If we use solar timing as a basis for defining seasons, we see that summer is the three months that have the greatest amount of solar radiation, and winter has the least. This puts the summer and winter solstices at the mid-point of the season. The beginning of each season will occur on the cross-quarter days. These are the days that are halfway between a solstice and an equinox. They do not occur on exactly the same date every year due to fluctuations in the relative orbits of earth, sun, and moon. For instance, the first day of spring will be near the beginning of February. In Chinese culture this is the merrily celebrated Chinese New Year, or Spring Festival. The cross-quarter day for the beginning of summer will be in the first week of May, for autumn it will fall around August 7, and winter will begin in the first week of November. Since solar energy is the basis of biology, this way of designating the seasons coincides with actual seasonal changes in light, temperature, and energy. The ideal schedule to follow when doing the practice of *Qigong Through the Seasons* would be to start Summer Qigong practice in early May, autumn in August, winter in November, and spring in February.

Modern Western science is beginning to research the importance of chronobiology to medical practice. The emerging field of *chronotherapy* studies how the timing of drug intake with medical procedures affects the therapeutic outcomes. In the past, patients were commonly instructed to take medication "once a day," often with little or no regard for what time of day or night. Current research has discovered that some drugs are more effective, and safer, if our circadian rhythms are taken into account.

Take for example, 5-fluorouracil (5-FU), which is used to treat colon cancer. This drug is now given at night when the cancer cells are more vulnerable and normal cells are resting and least sensitive. Also, the notorious morning pain from rheumatoid arthritis used to be treated with morning medications; however it has been found that if anti-inflammatory drugs are taken in the evening, they have fewer side-effects and are more effective for morning pain relief. Osteoarthritis is different than rheumatoid, with the worse pain coming in late afternoon or evening; for this type of arthritis many patients benefit most when they take pain medication at midday. Treatment regimens for other problems such as asthma, angina, hypertension, and psoriasis have also shown better results if the circadian rhythms of those diseases are considered in the treatment plan.

Cancer researchers are now pursuing further studies into the relationship between time and drug therapy. This burgeoning new field holds great promise for a more effective and humane treatment of people with cancer and other serious illnesses. However, the venerable wisdom tradition of China has, for thousands of years, recommended that not only should medical treatment be timed to innate cycles, but also the practices of qigong, meditation, and food therapy be linked to the daily, monthly, and yearly cycles of nature.

SEASONAL CYCLES

Now, go back to your wrist and feel the pulse again. It has more detailed information besides the number of beats per minute. A highly skilled practitioner of pulse diagnosis will be able to detect changes within the interior body through the subtle traits of the six major pulses (three on each wrist). Physiological dysfunctions or disease can often be recognized by the texture, amplitude, rhythm, width, and strength of the pulse at the radial artery. A healthy person will also, as explained in the classic texts of Chinese medicine, have some pulse variations that naturally coincide with the four major seasons of the year:

> In spring the pulse is slightly wiry, like the ripple or crest of a wave created by a fish swimming in a stream. The summer pulse is flooding and appears big near at the skin level. This is more like the surging waves in the ocean. The autumn pulse is just beneath the skin, as if insects are preparing their homes for winter. The winter pulse is deep and to the bone, as if an animal were hibernating in a cave. (Ni 1995, p.65)

The interaction between yin and yang essentially determines our health. The seasons are created by the ceaseless interplay of these two primordial powers: hot–cold, dry–wet, wind–calm, light–dark, all have critical influences on the planet's organic life. Therefore, if we truly want to be naturally healthy we will adjust our lifestyle to be in harmony with the yin–yang changes of nature. According to the Yellow Emperor, well-being comes from wisdom:

> The change of yin and yang through the four seasons is the root of life, growth, reproduction, aging, and destruction. By respecting this natural law it is possible to be free from illness. The sages have followed this, and the foolish people have not. (Ni 1995, p.7)

Spring and summer are the seasons when the Yang Qi builds up to it maximum strength, culminating at the Summer Solstice. Autumn and winter are the times when the Yin Qi predominates until the Winter Solstice. Some disorders occur more often in yang months, some more in yin months. Symptoms of ulcerative colitis, Crohn's disease, diabetes, and migraine headaches are worse during the yang phase of the year. Many mental health problems—anxiety, attention deficit hyperactivity disorder (ADHD), bipolar, schizophrenia, and obsessive/compulsive disorder—are more problematic in the yin phase. The peak month for episodic atrial fibrillation in the northern hemisphere is December. Testicular cancer most often gets diagnosed in winter. Cancerous breast lumps are most commonly detected in spring. Why is this so?

Some of these correlations are easy to explain from the single-cause perspective of Western science such as seasonal affective disorder (SAD). This malady occurs more often in winter because it usually directly relates to the number of daylight hours. But Western medicine has a harder time explaining how the detection of breast cancer is linked to the spring. Chinese medicine takes a broader view of human health. It does accept that SAD and winter are closely connected by daylight. But why do breast lumps appear more frequently during the Wood Phase of spring? The answer may be that spring is the time when the Yang Qi normally moves up from the lower body and into the chest. There it may encounter those formative cells that could become cancerous in almost any woman. But in this case, there is also stagnation of blood flow in the breast, which, when coupled with an influx of energy, could lead to a proliferation of quickly developing cancer cells.

Would you rather be a sage or a fool? Would you like to live in peace and harmony with nature, or do you think you can disregard natural law and still be free from illness? Are you interested in gaining access to the most powerful healing energy in the world, or are you going to settle for the hasty interventions of man-made therapies? Rather than relying on unnatural allopathic methods to treat these seasonally predisposed disorders, we can use qigong, meditation, and diet to strengthen the innate healing power within us and harmonize it with the prevailing healing energy of the seasons.

Spring

Wood Phase

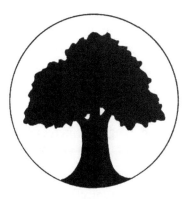

Spring relates to the Wood Phase—a heady, invigorating, sometimes disturbing season with wild fluctuations of energy surging throughout nature as birth, arousal, and movement. The momentum created by Spring Qi gives structure and impetus to the world: young trees thrusting skyward, icy rivers flooding valleys, babies everywhere screeching with the joy of life. In humans, qi rises like a slow tide coming up from its winter storage in the lower abdomen and moving into the chest where it stimulates the Liver with fresh vitality. As an infusion of energy, the Rising Qi carries benefits as well as the potential for problems. The practice of Spring Qigong centers on using qigong exercises, foods, and herbs, and meditation to nourish the Liver. In this chapter, you will learn how the Liver Network influences anger, kindness, communication, muscle function, detoxification, blood circulation, and much more.

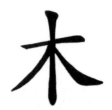

Figure 6.1: Wood character

The character for wood (Figure 6.1) depicts a tree. The image conveys a feeling of stability and verticality, a fitting description of good, healthy Spring Qi. Upward moving energy, whether in trees or humans, displays a statuesque posture that presents a sense of virility, competence, and durability. In people, the ascending yang energy imparts bodily strength and mental decisiveness. The wood character also has graceful downward sweeping lines, a definite yin attribute, which can be interpreted as lower branches or as roots extending underground. Altogether, this Chinese character beautifully presents a bold presence and a rooted foundation: a harmonious yin–yang picture of vibrant spring energy.

During spring, the Rising Yang Qi emerges from the LDT and begins a season-long ascent to the upper and outer regions of the body. As it passes into the MDT, it encounters the Liver. If this blood-rich organ retains stagnant blood and metabolic waste, which typically happens after winter's inactivity, it will obstruct the qi flow and result in Stagnant Liver Qi and Blood. According to Chinese medicine, the Liver controls the smooth and harmonious flow of qi and blood. Any obstruction to this flow will cause a serious functional disruption in qi and blood circulation. Stagnant Liver Qi and Blood, an all too common disorder, has physical symptoms of muscle pain, menstrual cramps, trembling movements, poor balance, headaches, neck pain, numbness in hands and feet, vision problems, digestive ailments, and more. The mental and emotional symptoms can run the spectrum from frustration and irritability to anger and rage.

LIVER NETWORK

The web of physical and mental correspondences relating to the Liver Network includes: Liver and gallbladder, muscles, tendons and fascia, eyes and sight, anger and kindness (see Table 2.1). If these diverse but interlinked elements are healthy and energetically balanced, you will stride through this season with vigor, ease, confidence, and determination.

Some people have an intrinsic structure and personality that identifies them as a "Wood type." A supple, muscular, and square physique with sinewy hands, strong slim feet, and a swarthy complexion are the traits of Wood. The person feels they have good balance with equal degrees of strength and flexibility. Wood types like to make choices and be competitive. Once they make a decision, they go for the goal with a direct and powerful commitment. Natural Wood types make good leaders when all these psychological tendencies are working in harmony. To other people they are obviously bold, assertive, and confident.

If these traits become exaggerated, or overactive, the person turns arrogant, compulsive, aggressive, confrontational, reckless, and tyrannical—they are not pleasant to be around. And they may abuse the use of stimulants and sedatives. Their volatile emotions and impatience can take them to disastrous extremes of behavior. If Wood types become overwrought, they may suffer from painful menses, premenstrual syndrome (PMS), high blood pressure, migraine headaches, occipital tension headaches, temporomandibular (TMJ) problems (the jaw joint in front of the ear), facial neuralgia (tics), tingling or numbness in the hands, and other disorders especially affecting the head and upper body.

Spring Qigong practice, which includes a recommended diet, will benefit the natural wood type by maintaining balance in their normal condition. And, definitely, this practice will help the exaggerated woody person by moderating their excessive tendencies. In the end, Spring Qigong will help everyone by nurturing Wood's positive qualities: curiosity, responsiveness, self-motivation, and expansion—wood wants to go forward.

ANGER, STAGNATION, AND KINDNESS

When the normal emotion of anger becomes prolonged, repressed, or inappropriate, it often results in Stagnant Liver Qi. This disorder affects women and men, but because each gender exists as fundamentally either yin or yang, qi stagnation usually results in different problems for each sex.

Men have innate yang energy; women have innate yin. Yang energy tends to expand outward; it's active and dispersive. Yin energy embraces receptivity, containment, and concentration. The gender predisposition to problems of Stagnant Liver Qi hinges on men being more yang/fire, and women more yin/blood. Stagnant Liver Qi, if not corrected, becomes virulent and flares up as Liver Fire in men and as Stagnant Liver Blood in women:

- *Anger > Stagnant Liver Qi + Men > "Liver Fire Rising" = muscle spasm, ulcers, hypertension, heart disease.*

- *Anger > Stagnant Liver Qi + Women > "Stagnant Liver Blood" = menstrual disorders, varicose veins, insomnia, anxiety.*

While disturbing and potentially dangerous, Stagnant Liver Qi can be effectively treated. Acupuncture and herbal remedies can release obstructions to the flow of qi and prevent stagnation. Qigong can remedy the condition by gathering fresh qi and properly circulating it through the body's energy pathways and storage centers. Meditation will definitely enhance qi flow, clear the mind of distractions, and nurture the virtue of kindness.

Numerous professional interventions can mitigate anger; however, each of us can learn to tame the beast through the practice of meditation and kindness. When we meditate on our feelings of anger, we can defuse an acute attack by mindfully investigating why we are angry at that moment. Does the feeling promote constructive or destructive change? How can we resolve it? With continued practice, meditation enables us to contemplate the deep background of anger and gain some insights into the origin of our suffering and what we must do to relieve it.

Kindness heals anger. Qigong master and scholar Kenneth Cohen states, "The anger of the liver is mended with kindness" (Cohen 1997, p.236). Each of the major organs has a positive attribute that promotes well-being. For the Liver it is *ren* or "human kindness"—the virtue that leads to acts of benevolence toward oneself and others. Confucius said, "Ren consists in loving others" (Analects XII, 22). Everyone in every culture would be better off if they would genuinely express kindness to one another. When a person consciously and sincerely offers kindness to those around him or her, the Liver can more easily promote the harmonious flow of qi and blood.

As a normal emotion, anger should be expressed like a lit match that burns brightly for a short time and then goes out. Anger is an agent of change. The *Chuang Tzu*, one of Daoism's sacred texts, illustrates the purpose of anger in the creation story of the Fish of the North.

> There was a great Fish in the ocean of the north, which is the origin of life. This great Fish rises from the sea to become a great Bird, representing the transformation of life from water to air. At the very moment of passage from the ocean to the air, the character for this effort of rising up is nu. This violent rising energy is not pathological; it is proper to all beginnings. (Larre and Rochat 1996, p.64)

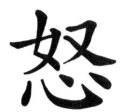

Figure 6.2: Anger character

The character for Anger is *nu* (Figure 6.2). The component on top signifies a female slave. It has two sides: the left side depicts a woman; the right side indicates a hand. The radical on the bottom means "HeartMind" or emotions (Schuessler 2007). All together, the word *nu* illustrates the emotions of a woman beneath the hand of a slave master with a general sense of "tension" (Schuessler 2007). The appearance of this character has the feeling of something about to explode or burst out of its subservient position, much like the energy of the great Fish when it became a great Bird.

Proper anger shows momentary passion and power; it should be like the burning match that flares brightly then fades away to be followed by appropriate action. It will have positive effects if it serves to achieve a worthwhile goal or to correct a wrong harmful to one self or others. This aspect of anger was the impetus behind the great Civil Rights Movement of the 1960s in the United States. But positive anger must be divorced from the wish to harm or destroy other people. Too often in our culture, anger turns into the extreme state of rage in which all rational thought vanishes with destructive rather than corrective outcomes.

HOW TO PRACTICE

All qigong practice sessions should begin with "Awakening the Qi" (see page 87) and should end with "Sealing the Qi" (see pages 96–7). This opening and closing will integrate body and mind with the energy centers and channels of qi circulation. Awakening the Qi serves as an energetic warm-up by stirring the LDT with your hands, calling to the UDT with your fingertips, and warming the Kidneys with massage. Sealing the Qi concludes the practice by bringing the energy back to the LDT. In this way you do not lose the wonderful health benefits just gained.

When you finish a qigong movement, do the "Cleansing Breath": Bring your feet together, stand with your arms relaxed down, your spine comfortably erect, and your eyes gazing softly into the distance. Take a deep inhalation, and then audibly and completely exhale through your mouth. Stand quietly for a few moments, intentionally point your fingers toward earth and feel the qi circulating through your body. Too often people will fidget around after doing a qigong exercise or rush into the next movement; this dissipates the energy just cultivated. The Cleansing Breath allows the qi to continue moving along the intended course, thus enhancing energy flow and mental equanimity. Most importantly, it brings you back to earth so that you remain rooted to this source of energy throughout the practice routine. It only takes a brief time to do, so do not neglect this important centering exercise.

Most styles of qigong have three aspects to every exercise: body movement, mental intention, and rhythmic breathing. These three factors have shifting proportions depending on the season. Spring Qigong highlights expansive and robust external body movements. While doing these exercises, be attentive to how your muscles work, take notice of any soreness or restrictions and how that changes with practice, and combine breathing and moving to expel turbid energy from the muscles and boost blood circulation. Put some effort (gong) into Spring Qigong and reap the rewards of smoothly flowing qi and blood.

SPRING QIGONG

> The Liver governs the smooth and harmonious flow of qi and blood.
>
> (*The Yellow Emperor's Classic of Medicine*)

Any disruption of vital blood and qi flow can result in muscle pain/cramps, erratic movements, joint stiffness, emotional irritability, and more. To correct these conditions we need to release any stagnation or obstructions of qi and blood in the Liver. These knots can be undone with qigong practice, acupuncture, and herbs. The Liver naturally opens to external influences—both good and bad—in springtime; therefore, we should take this opportunity to positively affect its health. Spring Qigong practice uses "external qigong" exercises that emphasize muscle movement, opening the chest and expelling stagnant qi from the MDT. The "internal qigong" exercise, Enhancing Liver Qi, effectively balances the yin and yang aspects of the Liver Network.

Do eight repetitions of each exercise unless otherwise noted.

Awakening the Qi

Lower Dan Tian

Use your right palm to rub 36 times clockwise around your navel. Then replace your right palm with your left and rub 36 times counterclockwise.

Beat the Heavenly Drum

Cover your ears with the heels of your hands. Then tap with the fingertips on your occipital bone for about 10 seconds.

Massage the Kidneys

Form loose fists with your hands, then massage up and down over your lower back 36 times.

Do Awakening the Qi only once.

Sunrise—Sunset

Stand with your feet hip-width apart. Bend over from your waist, let your hands hang down toward the floor (Figure 6.3). Interlace your fingers so your palms are facing your head. Your fingers remain interlaced throughout the entire exercise.

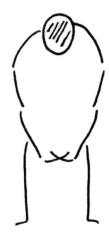

Figure 6.3: Sunrise—Sunset

Inhale as you straighten up. Lift your hands close to your body, turn them over at chest level, and raise your arms overhead (Figure 6.4). Lift your heels off the floor, palms facing heaven.

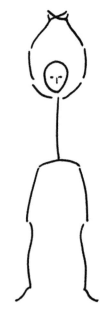

Figure 6.4: Sunrise—Sunset

Exhale as you return your heels to the floor. Bend over at the waist, keeping your arms/elbows straight as you bring your hands down toward your feet, then turn the palms toward your head. That is one repetition.

Visualize bringing energy up from the earth, through your body, and up to heaven.

Spinal Cord Breathing

Stand with your feet shoulder-width apart, and your hands at your sides.

Inhale as you bring your hands up to ear level, with the fingers spread wide and palms facing forward (Figure 6.5). Your upper arms are at 45 degrees, and your forearms are vertical. At the same time, pull your shoulders back and tilt your head back. Your sacrum is thrust backward, and your full spine is in extension.

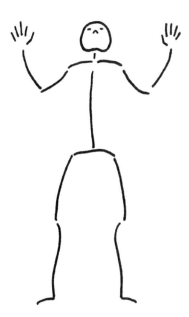

Figure 6.5: Spinal Cord Breathing

Exhale loudly as your spine goes into flexion. Bring your forearms together, forming your hands in fists (Figure 6.6). Your elbows press into your ribs, your chin is tucked into your chest, and your hips are curled under. That is one repetition.

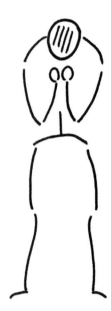

Figure 6.6: Spinal Cord Breathing

Visualize the chest opening and closing, the spine fully extending and flexing. Begin slowly, and then pick up the pace a little. Always exhale forcefully through your mouth.

Press Back to Banish all Illness

Stand with your feet close together, your arms crossed at the wrists with your hands open and your palms against your chest (Figure 6.7). Step forward with your right foot and place the toes lightly on the floor, keeping your weight on your left leg.

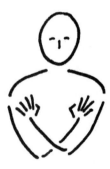

Figure 6.7: Press Back to Banish all Illness

Inhale as you turn your body to the right while pressing forward with your left palm and backward with your right palm, looking over your right hand (Figure 6.8). All fingers are pointing upward.

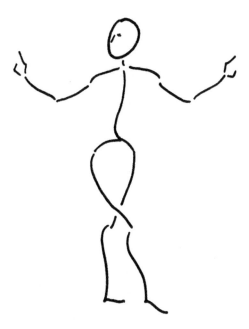

Figure 6.8: Press Back to Banish all Illness

Exhale and return to the starting position, with arms crossed. Step forward with your left foot and place the toes lightly on the floor. Keep your weight on your right leg with the knee bent. That is one repetition.

Inhale as you turn your body to the left while pressing forward with your right palm and backward with your left palm, looking over your left hand. All fingers are pointing upward.

Exhale and return to the starting position, with arms crossed. Step forward with your right foot and place the toes lightly on the floor. Keep your weight on your left leg with the knee bent. That is the second repetition.

Visualize rotating on the spinal axis, opening and closing the chest.

Shoot the Bow

Stand with your feet together, and your hands at your sides.

Inhale as you bring your palms together in the prayer position at chest level (Figure 6.9). Bend both knees slightly.

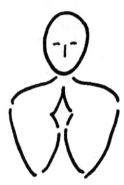

Figure 6.9: Shoot the Bow

Exhale loudly as you step to the side with your right foot, toes pointing to the right (Figure 6.10). Your weight shifts to your right leg. Your left palm lightly slaps your ribcage on your right side. Your right hand extends to the right with the index finger pointing to the right. Look over the pointing finger. This is one repetition.

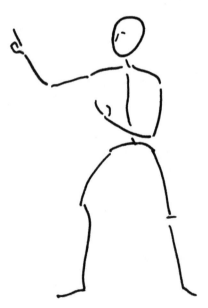

Figure 6.10: Shoot the Bow

Inhale as you step back to the center. Straighten your knees, and circle both hands down and then up to prayer position. Then bend both knees.

Exhale loudly as you step to the side with your left foot. Your weight shifts to your left leg. Slap your left ribs with your right palm, point and look over your left finger. This is the second repetition.

Visualize expelling stagnant qi from the MDT.

Enhancing Liver Qi

The three basic ingredients of qigong—movement, breathing, and intention—come into play equally in this potent exercise. The hand/arm *movements* bring healing qi from the environment into the three *dan tians*; then the hands gather and store more qi into the MDT; and finally the *laogong* points in the palms make a rooted connection between the earth and you. *Laogong* functions as the most powerful acupuncture point on the human body for projecting and receiving qi. The *breathing* component of this qigong exercise manifests as the healing sounds. These sacred vocalizations synchronize with the downward movement of the hands to resonate with the three energy centers, causing an infusion of acoustic qi specific to that region of the body. *Intention*, in step with the moving hands, brings energy down the *Taiji Axis* to augment the *dan tians*. Intention also packs qi into the MDT and the Liver through the *qimen* point. *Qimen* is located on the bottom edge of the ribcage at a hand's width distance from the midline of the torso. According to the textbooks from the Shanghai College of Traditional Medicine, stimulation of *qimen* "facilitates the spreading of Liver Qi, transforms and removes Congealed Blood" (O'Connor and Bensky 1985). Enhancing Liver Qi reigns as one of the best exercises for relaxing and opening up the Liver, expediting qi flow through the *Taiji Axis*, and settling the mind in the body.

Begin by standing with your feet hip-width apart, and your hands down at your sides.

Inhale and raise your arms out to the sides, then overhead to bring your palms together (Figure 6.11).

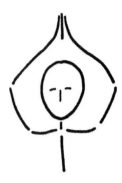

Figure 6.11: Enhancing Liver Qi

Exhale and begin to bring your praying hands down in front (Figure 6.12). Vocalize OM as your hands slowly pass by your head; then AH as they pass your throat; and then HUN (hoon) at your chest as your hands turn over with the fingers pointing down. Continue exhaling and lower your hands to the LDT. The three-syllable sound has an even tone until the end of "hoon," where the pitch slightly drops. Finish the exhalation with your palms together and fingers pointing down at the level of the LDT.

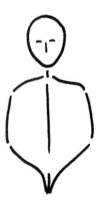

Figure 6.12: Enhancing Liver Qi

Inhale as your hands separate and move forward at chest level with the palms facing each other.

Exhale as you bring your hands back until your elbows are near your ribs and your shoulders are relaxed (Figure 6.13). Hold your hands there and *take three breaths. Feel the movement in the MDT and ribs:* the hands move slightly apart with the inhalation and come within inches of each other on the exhalation.

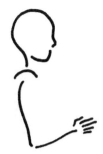

Figure 6.13: Enhancing Liver Qi

Inhale as your hands make a scooping action toward the back (Figure 6.14), then finish inhaling as the palms turn up and the little fingers touch the edge of the lower ribs (Figure 6.15).

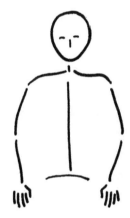

Figure 6.14: Enhancing Liver Qi

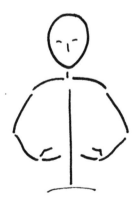

Figure 6.15: Enhancing Liver Qi

Exhale, relax, and *think of sending qi from your hands into your body through the qimen point*. Hold that position for one breath, *inhale* and *exhale*.

Then *inhale* again.

Exhale as you press your elbows against your ribs, then move your hands forward with the palms up to chest level. *Think of squeezing out turbid qi from the body*. Finish exhaling as the palms turn down and your forearms are parallel to the ground. Your index fingers are slightly elevated above the other fingers (Figure 6.16).

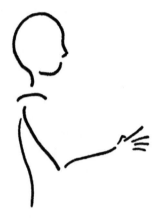

Figure 6.16: Enhancing Liver Qi

Relax and stay in this position for *three breaths*. Feel that the *laogong* points are anchored to the earth, the whole body is strong, the MDT spacious. *Think of energy connecting the laogong points with the earth*.

Do Enhancing Liver Qi three times.

Sealing the Qi

Whole Body Tapping

Use your palms to tap over each arm, your trunk, outer legs, inner legs, abdomen, lower back (use your fists on your back). Do this three times.

Arms Horizontal

Put your arms straight out to the sides, with your fingers pointing up, for one breath.

Heaven and Earth

Inhale and lift your hands laterally and then overhead, with the palms pointing to heaven. Rise up on your toes and hold your breath for a few seconds. Slowly exhale, lower your heels, and with palms facing the earth, lower your hands to the LDT.

Seal

Cover the LDT with the palm of your right hand. Place the palm of your left hand over your right hand with the thumb tucked under your right hand. Stand quietly for three breaths.

Do Sealing the Qi only once.

NEIGONG PRACTICE—ENTERING TRANQUILITY

Internal qigong and meditation often blend together in the practice of *Qigong Through the Seasons.* They both nourish qi in all of its yin–yang manifestations—abiding in tranquility or freely circulating—by using inwardly directed intention and visualization. Inner Nourishing and Rising Yang Qi exemplify this fusion of qigong and meditation.

Releasing unwanted tightness around the internal organs can be achieved with deep qigong practice. Qi can only circulate with maximum efficiency and greatest value when no excessive tension exists in the organs, the surrounding muscles, the web of connective tissue, or the intrinsic vessels and nerves. Physiological tranquility, gained from qigong practice, feels like an alert peacefulness melding the body and mind together into a complete whole. Dr. Jiao Guorui, a highly respected twentieth-century qigong practitioner in China, calls this state "entering quiescence" (Jiao 1990, p.61). He describes it as a major requirement for practice:

> First of all, we must understand the quiescent state correctly. This state exists relatively as compared to the dynamic state. Life is movement, and the quiescent state is actually stillness in movement. It is not motionless. Therefore, qigong exercise is essentially quiescent motions. When we enter the quiescent state we are entering a special state of movement. (Jiao 1990, p.61)

Dr. Jiao refers to the movement of qi. What signifies quiescence? Think of it as a special state of inward tranquility, composure, and rest. For some people, entering tranquility feels like a frozen river that melts during springtime, thereby releasing stagnated energy, pent-up emotions, and mental dismay. Mental and emotional tranquility eliminates interferences from both inside and outside the body, providing favorable conditions for the central nervous system to carry out the active, natural regulation of body functions and cognitive abilities.

The condition of being "completely relaxed" allows the Liver to perform its myriad tasks with unfettered power. This amazing visceral structure has more functions that any other single organ: it filters and detoxifies the blood, produces hundreds of enzymes and hormones, and regulates the volume of circulating blood. Oftentimes, due to poor diet, stress, irritability, and inactivity, the Liver becomes clogged and sluggish. For this vital organ to work properly, it must become decongested and supple. The Chinese say that a healthy Liver resembles "a Free and Easy Wanderer," responsible for the smooth and harmonious flow of blood and qi throughout the body and mind.

During spring, the concentration of qi rises up from the Kidney area and pours into the MDT. At this point, if congealed metabolic waste products clog the Liver, the Rising Qi will become trapped, thus causing Stagnated Liver Qi and Blood (more about this later in the chapter). Spring Qigong practice helps the Liver become free and easy through the use of special qigong exercises, herbs, and foods. The following practice, Inner Nourishing, combines internal qigong practice together with meditation to create whole person tranquility, thus relaxing the Liver and freeing the flow of qi.

Inner Nourishing

Inner Nourishing, *Nei Yang Gong*, developed as a secret Daoist healing method during the Ming dynasty; qigong masters traditionally transmitted it to only one select student. In 1947 Dr. Liu Guizhen, feeling that everyone should know this health-enhancing internal practice for the greater good of society, began to teach it to the public. Inner Nourishing exemplifies how *neigong* and meditation merge into a single practice through the combination of breathing, movement, mindfulness, and visualization.

Begin by sitting or lying down (Figure 6.17). Rest and be comfortable but alert.

Inhale slowly and think of bringing the qi from the tailbone area, up your back, over your head and into your mouth. While inhaling gently, place the tip of your tongue on the roof of your mouth just behind the front teeth, and silently say, "I am calm."

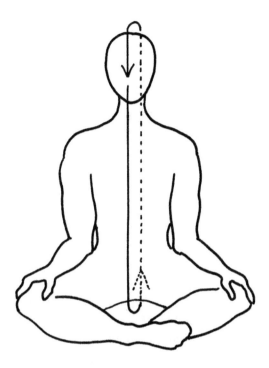

Figure 6.17: Inner Nourishing

Exhale slowly and think of bringing the qi down the front of your body to the LDT. While exhaling, let your tongue drop gently to the floor of your mouth as you silently say, "and relaxed."

Do this for a few minutes. Don't count repetitions; just breathe slowly, visualize energy moving up your back and down your front in harmony with the silent mantra. This meditative practice not only moves the qi up the Governing Meridian and down the Conception Meridian, it effectively elicits a deep relaxation response throughout the entire body. You can even do this while sitting at work, in an airplane or bus, or standing in a line waiting for something to happen.

Progressive Relaxation

The practice of Progressive Relaxation serves as muscle therapy. While not a classical qigong exercise, since it does not focus on qi movement, it can be part of any qigong practice or meditation session at any season or phase of the year. It works well as a link between moving and sitting. Due to its emphasis on muscle function, Progressive Relaxation is especially appropriate for the Liver Network when the muscles and tendons are most involved. And since irritability and stress are often prevalent during spring, Progressive Relaxation will also help with those conditions.

Good health depends in part on the ability to completely relax tight muscles. The accumulation of tension in any tissue impedes blood and qi circulation, which leads to a toxic build-up of metabolic debris resulting in achiness, stiffness, and outright pain. Sustained muscle discomfort eventually produces a cloud of anxiety and edginess, eventually causing a spectrum of symptoms from constipation to headaches. If you can consciously release muscular tension, your health status will be greatly improved. As you have learned, the Liver controls the smooth flow of qi and blood. Anxiety, anger, and impaired movement of Rising Yang Qi in the spring can cause obstructions to this normal flow, resulting in the unwanted condition of Stagnant Liver Qi and Blood.

Many researchers have studied the body's reactions to meditation, qigong, muscular relaxation, and various types of regulated breathing techniques. These methods have some common benefits that include lowered blood pressure, decreased tension in muscles, reduction of stress hormones in the blood, and induction of alpha brain waves signaling calmness. Together, these benefits constitute what has come to be known as the "relaxation response."

Progressive Relaxation can provide a very effective method for eliminating undue muscular tension. This technique proceeds by systematically tensing and then relaxing certain muscle groups in a sequence going from your feet to your head. By breathing mindfully during this Progressive Relaxation, you can achieve all the benefits of the deep relaxation response.

Begin by lying down comfortably on your back where you can place your hands by your sides with the palms up.

Inhale as you flex your *ankles* and strongly pull your toes toward your chest for about 3–4 seconds. Then *exhale* and completely relax your feet as you let go of all tension. Pause for three more slow, gentle breaths without any muscular contractions. Then move your awareness up to the hip area.

Inhale deeply as you squeeze your *buttocks* together for 3–4 seconds. Notice how your pelvis rises up…then release your hips as you *exhale*. Completely relax the whole pelvic area inside and out. Take at least three slow breaths in compete relaxation. Now move your awareness up to your shoulder blades.

Inhale as you take a deep breath in and pull your *shoulder blades* together for 3–4 seconds. Notice how your chest rises up…now *exhale* and mindfully relax your upper back and chest completely. Again, take three or more easy breaths. Feel your body resting comfortably on the floor. Move your awareness down your arms to your hands.

Inhale as you clench your *hands* into tight fists for 3–4 seconds. Feel your forearms tense and your hands tighten. Then *exhale* and purposefully straighten out the fingers so that the *laogong* points in the palms are open. Then let the fingers rest back into their naturally curled neutral position. Again, take three breaths. Then move your awareness to the top of your shoulders.

Inhale as you pull your *shoulders* toward your ears. Really squeeze them upward. *Exhale* and completely relax your shoulders. You may want to slightly pull them back down to a resting state. Take three breaths and feel how your upper back is open and resting comfortably on the floor. Take a few more relaxing breaths. Finally, move your awareness to your face.

Inhale and squeeze all the *face* muscles together into a pucker. *Exhale* and mindfully, completely, relax your entire face. Relax your neck and let your head rest comfortably on the floor. Now, enjoy the serenity you have just created with Progressive Relaxation.

SPRING MEDITATION
Rising Yang Qi Meditation

This meditation will show you how to use the Yang Qi, the great activating energy of nature, for spiritual awakening. Yang Qi physically causes the movement of our internal organs, the upward growth of a young plant, the fiery radiation of the sun. Mentally, Yang Qi gives us the power of rational thinking and analysis. Spiritually, this inspiring energy illuminates the path that can take us beyond the limits of body and mind. In its highest evolutionary form, Yang Qi turns into *Shen*—the spiritual energy that completes our life. You are going to direct the qi up the *Taiji Axis*, through the three *dan tians*, and out into the world (see Figure 6.18). Please note that the following instructions give general guidelines for time at each *dan tian*; but you may stay at any center for as long as you want.

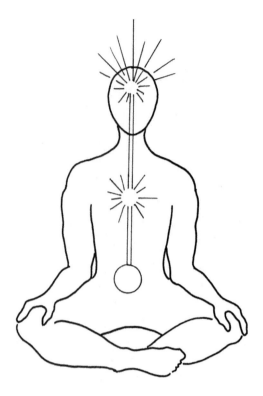

Figure 6.18: Rising Yang Qi

Begin by sitting on a cushion or chair. Put your attention on the LDT. Let your mind and your breath rest there. Let your abdomen relax. Let your lower back relax. Look inward.

Visualize a small ball of yellow light in the middle of the LDT. Breathe into this area. Feel that your breath motivates this light. Bringing it to life, giving it movement and creating warmth. As you breathe slowly…peacefully…feel the warmth from this yellow ball of light spreading throughout your lower abdomen. Relax into the warm yellow glow for a few minutes.

And now, bring this light very slowly up through the *Taiji Axis. The ball now becomes a beam of light*—like a column of mercury rising in a thermometer. Spend a couple of minutes slowly bringing this beam of light from the LDT up through your intestines and stomach toward your chest. Nourish the area with your breath as if you were blowing on a hot coal, making more heat.

This yellow light comes into the MDT and mixes with the blood red color of the Heart. Yellow turns a deep *reddish-gold*. Feel it warm and relax the entire area of your chest. The column of light has lost its shape. It's just pure light without a form or structure. Now the space around your Heart and Liver glows with a beautiful reddish-gold color. Let your attention dwell in the MDT, in a vibrant cloud of color, for a few more minutes. Feel a subtle, slow pulsing of light, as if the light itself were breathing.

Now, use your intention to *bring this light upward into your head*. It is as if your mind is beckoning this energy into the UDT at the center of your brain—the abode of the *Shen*, the human Spirit. The light becomes brighter as it fills this spiritual palace. Breathe softly and see the colored light changing into a white luminescence inflating the UDT with a sense of love and benevolence. Begin to release this spiritual energy from the confines of your body.

The energy now extends out through the top of your head, like rays from a rising sun, fanning out in all directions. Just breathe comfortably. Feel this Rising Yang Qi coming up through your body and expanding out everywhere, touching everything in your environment, rising upward to the sky, becoming as limitless as the sky itself.

The light no longer has a color. Only pure Yang Qi. Feel that your whole body emanates this energy, becoming a part of each facet in the jewel of creation. Your whole body is breathing, radiating energy. As you sit and breathe comfortably, let all thoughts of the past and desires for the future fade into the distance. Let go of bodily boundaries—be just light. Let go of time.

Now the Yang Qi has transformed into the Shen and your Spirit blends with the consciousness of nature. Just breathe quietly. Let yourself rest in this primordial stillness and you will realize an intimacy with all things; the true awakening of the human Spirit.

Finish by sitting like this for a few more minutes. Let your body and your mind fill the great limitless space around you.

SUGGESTIONS FOR SPRING PRACTICE

You may combine qigong exercises and the meditations in various ways to develop your personal practice routine. My daily work schedule varies so that sometimes I only have 10–15 minutes to practice, whereas on other days I can devote time to a longer session. The exercises and meditation may be grouped in many different ways. Here are some suggestions for a short qigong session:

1. Awakening the Qi; Sunrise–Sunset; Spinal Cord Breathing; Shoot the Bow; Enhancing Liver Qi; Sealing the Qi. *Cultivates physical conditioning and qi circulation.*

2. Awakening the Qi; Spinal Cord Breathing; Press Back to Banish all Illness; Sealing the Qi; Enhancing Liver Qi; Inner Nourishing; Sealing the Qi. *Cultivates qi in the MDT.*

3. Awakening the Qi; Sunrise–Sunset; Enhancing Liver Qi; Inner Nourishing; Sealing the Qi. *Cultivates Liver Qi.*

A complete session will include all of the qigong exercises done in the order presented in this chapter. I do the long practice at least three times a week. Progressive Relaxation can be done independently or fit into any of the above groups. I like to do it in the evening as the day settles into night. The nature of Rising Yang Qi meditation makes it a perfect morning practice. But, of course, any time you meditate is a good time to meditate. Take all of this information and make it your own; experiment with various groupings; notice how certain groups are internally or externally biased. Although traditionally practiced in the morning, you should develop a routine where practice fits in with the rest of your schedule. Don't let it become a source of conflict; but don't neglect it either.

FOOD, FLAVORS, AND HERBS FOR SPRING

Green, upward growing vegetables provide the Rising Yang Qi that begins to move during the Wood Phase. Eating these foods—asparagus tops the list—adds a healthy dose of active energy to your body. Other foods that embody the Rising Yang Qi are celery, bok choy, romaine lettuce, and all the leafy vegetables that grow toward the sun. In addition to the upward reaching foods, sprouting seeds have enormous quantities of qi for the purpose of pushing up into the light. Add sprouts to your diet and you will take in that same vitality, along with a good dose of B vitamins and enzymes that facilitate digestion.

The *sour* flavor dynamically influences the Liver Network: its astringent contracting action releases stagnation from the Liver and moves qi upward. Sourness also assists in the digestion of fatty foods and proteins. Beyond being good for the Liver, the sour flavor can be used to treat conditions of flaccidity and leakage: diarrhea, hemorrhoids, uterine or rectal prolapse, and urinary incontinence. This is a yin flavor, so you should not overdo it in the Rising Yang Qi season. For example, you can safely drink the

Lemon Liver Cleanser (see page 106) three to four times a week; this will give you an excellent yin–sour tonic to balance the burgeoning Yang Qi, but doing it every day may cause too much contraction. Excellent sources for the sour flavor are rhubarb, vinegar, citrus fruits, yogurt, pickles, and sauerkraut.

The following foods and herbs also have particular effects on the Liver:

- *Relax the Liver and move the qi:*
  - asparagus
  - bupleurum
  - cabbage
  - lemon, basil
  - black pepper
  - cayenne
  - celery
  - coconut milk
  - dill
  - garlic
  - ginger
  - safflower oil.

- *Detoxify the Liver and purify the blood:*
  - dandelion
  - milk thistle
  - bupleurum
  - alfalfa
  - echinacea
  - angelica
  - yarrow
  - ginseng.

—————— Lemon Liver Cleanser ——————

Many cultures use this beverage as an excellent spring tonic. Drink it 2–4 times a week. Mix 1 tbsp of pure maple syrup, the juice of one lemon, and a pinch of cayenne pepper into 8 fl oz (236ml) of warm water. Stir to blend the syrup and water, then drink and enjoy.

While we should increase our consumption of sprouting seeds, young greens, and other seasonal foods in spring, we should also eat those herbs and foods that have been shown to stimulate the flow of Liver Qi and detoxify the blood, regardless of the season.

Herbs for Spring

We have seen how Stagnant Liver Qi can be extremely upsetting both to the person who suffers from it and for the people in their proximity. Skeletal muscle tension, tightness around the ribcage, generalized irritability, dizziness, neck pain, and dull headaches usually indicate a moderate form of this disorder. When fully blown up, Stagnant Liver Qi will cause menstrual cramps, inappropriate anger or rage, stabbing muscle pain, hypertension, pain or bloating in the upper digestive tract, and more. Unfortunately, sluggish qi and blood occurs frequently in our culture due to eating foods that clog the Liver, lack of muscular exercise, and perhaps most of all, unrelenting stress. However, Stagnant Liver Qi was also a problem thousands of years ago in China where pent-up emotions, servitude, and malnutrition would shut down the free flow of qi and blood, resulting in the signs and symptoms mentioned above.

Chinese doctors, through generations of research, formulated an herbal combination that proved very effective in treating blocked energy and stale blood, which in turn would calm the Spirit and improve digestion. This famous formula is *xiao yao san*, commonly translated as Free and Easy Wanderer. Of all the herbal tonics that I use in my clinic, this one is the most frequently prescribed because of its effectiveness for Stagnant Liver Qi and Blood. Besides relieving primary symptoms of muscle pain/cramps, tension, and headaches, patients often report that their bowel function has improved and they feel more relaxed. The chief herbs in *xiao yao san* are bupleurum (*chai hu*), angelica (*dang gui*), and peony (*bai shao*); a choice of synergistic herbs are added to this base to address the patient's specific condition.

Bupleurum is a bitter herb that, like the sour flavor, will cleanse the Liver of metabolic waste and stagnant blood; this action releases heat from the Liver, thus soothing emotions and cooling the internal environment. Bupleurum moves qi higher in the body, making it compatible with the natural Rising Yang Qi of spring; this upward lifting action also helps relieve prolapse of some tissues, especially the bladder and hemorrhoids.

Angelica sinensis is well known by its Chinese name, *dang gui*. Gratefully used by women around the world for PMS and dysmenorrhea, *dang gui* supplements and invigorates blood throughout the body making it appropriate for any woman or man who has trouble with tight, sore muscles, general lassitude, and sluggish bowels. Different parts of the plant are used for different conditions, so you should consult with a knowledgeable herbalist before using; in that way your formula will be most beneficial and safe.

Peony (*bai shao*) functions much like bupleurum for relieving cramps and moving the blood, but it tends to work more on the emotional aspect of Stagnant Liver Qi. White Peony tonifies the Yin Qi everywhere in the body and mind, giving more internal strength to people with frail and cold conditions. Like bupleurum and angelica, *bai shao* releases blood congestion and frees the qi; it especially helps to soothe the irascibility and moodiness caused by Liver congestion.

If, after reading this information on the Liver Network and the symptoms of Stagnant Liver Qi, you suspect that your Liver could benefit from herbal therapy, please seek a professional consultant. The proper diagnosis and subsequent recommendations will ensure that your herbal medicine will be safe and successful in relieving your suffering. You should first emphasize natural season-specific foods and doing the Spring Qigong practice to stay healthy; then, if symptoms suggest the need for further treatment, talk to a licensed practitioner for advice.

RECIPES FOR SPRING

Asparagus Tips

(Serves 4–6 as a side dish)

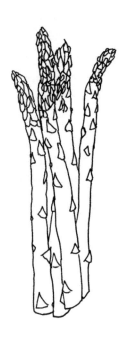

1 tbsp sesame seeds

¼ cup cashews

2 tbsp sesame oil

2 lb (1 kg) asparagus, trimmed to the top
2 inches of each spear—just the "tips"

1 tbsp soy sauce

1 scallion, with white bulb and 3 inches of
green, thinly sliced

Heat a small, dry, heavy skillet on medium high. When the skillet is hot add the sesame
seeds and heat until just starting to brown. Be careful, they brown quickly. Remove from

the skillet and set aside. Wipe the skillet, then add the cashews and heat until they start to turn brown. Stir frequently. Remove from the skillet and set aside.

Heat the sesame oil in a wok or large skillet until quite hot, but not smoking—be careful not to burn the oil.

Add the asparagus tips and cook over medium heat, tossing frequently, for 3 minutes. Add the soy sauce, sesame seeds, and cashews. Cook over a medium-high heat for another 2 minutes.

Garnish with the sliced scallions and serve immediately.

Rhubarb Bread

(Makes one 9 x 4 inches loaf)

2 cups flour	2 tbsp melted butter
½ tsp salt	Boiling water
1½ tsp baking powder	1 egg, beaten
½ tsp baking soda	1 cup chopped pecans
1 cup sugar	1 cup chopped fresh raw rhubarb
Juice and zest of 1 organic orange	

Preheat the oven to 325°F (160°C/Gasmark 3). Grease bottom of a loaf pan.

Sift the flour and other dry ingredients into a large mixing bowl.

In a 1-cup measure, mix the orange juice and melted butter; fill with boiling water to measure 1 cup.

Add to the dry ingredients along with the beaten egg and stir to mix completely. Fold in the pecans and rhubarb.

Pour into the prepared loaf pan, and bake for about 75 minutes.

Remove from the oven and let the bread cool in the pan for about 10 minutes. Then remove from the pan and allow to cool completely before slicing.

Asparagus and Salmon

(Serves 4)

4 salmon fillets

1 tsp dried rosemary

½ tsp ground black pepper, divided

14 fl oz (400g) vegetable broth

juice of one lemon

8 oz (225g) fresh asparagus, trimmed and cut into 2-inch pieces

Season the salmon with the rosemary and ¼ tsp pepper. Place in a large skillet.

In a small bowl, combine the broth, lemon juice, and the remaining ¼ tsp pepper; mix well and pour into the skillet with the fish.

Cover and bring to a boil over medium heat, then reduce the heat to low and simmer for 5 minutes.

Place the asparagus around the salmon, then cover and cook for 5 more minutes, or until the fish flakes easily and the asparagus is tender.

Serve immediately.

WHEN DOES SPRING ACTUALLY BEGIN?

Our standard Gregorian calendar says that spring begins in the northern hemisphere on the Vernal Equinox, around March 20, when the sun shines directly over the equator at noon. But for meteorologists, each season begins at the first of the respective months—March 1 for the spring season. Then there were the ancient Celtic and Germanic people who celebrated the first day of spring around the beginning of February on the "cross-quarter day" located at that mid-point between the last solstice and the next equinox (this then makes March 20 the middle of spring). China celebrates its most important holiday, the Spring Festival, between the end of January and middle of February. Different cultures have different ways to designate seasons, but they are just man-made selections. So how do we know when spring has actually sprung?

When in doubt, always look to nature for the answers. When we see budding new leaves on plants we take it as a sure sign that spring has begun. We usually think that longer hours of daylight and/or warming temperatures determine this new growth. But do they?

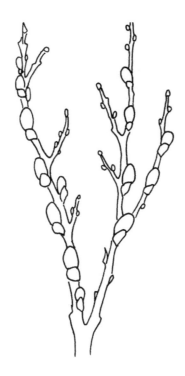

I have a lovely elm bonsai tree. It is about the size of a soccer ball and lives in a round ceramic pot. Like all deciduous trees, this elm needs a dormant period to rest but it can't tolerate prolonged freezing. So I put it in a small, dark closet attached to the outside of the house where the temperature stays around 40°F (4°C) degrees. Every February I look forward to a miracle. This little tree, which has spent the winter in total darkness and at a constant temperature, begins to come alive with a multitude of new leaves in the first half of February. When I peer into the dim light of the opened closet and see little drops of green all over the bonsai tree, I know that spring has arrived.

What causes this tree to bud out? As you have seen, it was not increasing periods of light or changing temperatures; those factors remained unchanged. What empowered this plant to break out of its dormancy and burst forth with the green promise of new growth? The answer: nature's Rising Yang Qi. This unstoppable force ascends throughout the northern hemisphere at this time of year, while the dominant Yin Qi of winter slowly wanes. The bonsai tree, just like every other living thing, irresistibly responds to the endless interchange of yin and yang. There is no other plausible explanation for what engendered the bud break on this tree while it was in total darkness. Think about this truly remarkable example of how strongly qi movement affects life.

Qi movement depends on the rise and demise of yin and yang; the cyclical movement of qi causes the seasons to change. Qi energy keeps all sentient beings alive on earth. Qi is the kinetic force that powers every type of movement in the cosmos, constantly ebbing and flowing between its two phases: yin and yang. The Yang Qi increases throughout the spring and reaches its zenith at the Summer Solstice. Then the Yang Qi begins to wane and the Yin Qi increasingly dominates the northern latitudes until the Winter Solstice.

We are part of nature. This essential seasonal movement of qi also occurs within us. Consider again the bonsai tree sleeping in complete darkness—what primal shift does it feel in its roots, how much energy must rise up the trunk to open the leaves? What sparked this transformation from yin to yang? There exists a mysterious power that you will never see, hear, touch, taste, or smell; nevertheless you are deeply affected by its unceasing presence during every moment of your life. Qigong practice shows you how to tap into this life-giving force and use it for your greater good.

Chapter 7

Summer

Fire Phase

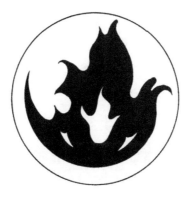

Summer energy urges us to get moving. We want to be outside more often, we wear fewer clothes, and are in closer contact with nature. We like to spend time in joyful physical recreation and gatherings with friends. Summer stimulates creativity, which we may express with building projects, designing gardens, making music, art objects, and party decorations—anything that gives us warm pleasurable connections to people and outdoors adventures. During this season of splendor and shining fire, the energy of nature grows outward with color, warmth, and radiance. Now our Spirit comes alive with expansive awareness; it wants to make intimate contact with all the elements of heaven and earth.

During the Fire Phase we feel that our Heart Qi, which was fueled by the Rising Yang Qi of spring, has come into full bloom with expressions of joy, compassion and a mysterious yearning for divine contact. The exuberance of Fire, when controlled and cultivated, can be refined and directed toward the ultimate purpose of being human: spiritual awakening. However—if not properly harnessed—the great blazing of summer's Supreme Yang Qi can scorch our Heart and mind. Summer Qigong practice will show you how to feed the *Heart Network* without getting burned.

The character for fire is *huo* (roughly "who wa"). The image depicts bright flames swooping upward to show that fire's essential nature ascends, spreads, and illuminates (Figure 7.1). At the same time, the broad base gives ample stability to the character, indicating that for fire to flame upward it must have plentiful fuel. All together this is a simple and well-balanced character that conveys the sense of a benign fire cooking food and keeping us warm.

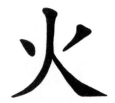

Figure 7.1: Fire character

The Fire Phase symbolizes maturity. Just as noon occurs at the zenith of daily yang energy, summer epitomizes the ultimate yang season—day and season shine high and bright at the apex of qi circulation. Early summer was filled with much heated activity due to the yang Qi's influence, but after the Summer Solstice the sun begins to lean toward the south and we have a sense of completion. We can now sit back and enjoy the fruits of our projects, the bounty of our gardens.

The energy of fire needs to be just right for it to be healthy. Fire should not be too hot. That degree of heat would boil away the body's water leaving us parched and brittle; mentally it would make us aggressive, interfering, and scattered. Everything about us would be excessive. Anxiety, insomnia, agitation, neurological disorders, and substance abuse are some of the signs of hyperactive fire. If we become stuck in this intemperate zone, we are not pleasant company: boundaries get pushed, the body overheats and bizarre behavior prevails. The actions that we intend to be joyful and intimate maybe perceived by others as frenzied and obsessed.

A good healthy fire feels "warm." It emanates from the Heart. It keeps us stable, flexible, and friendly such that we project a comforting presence of body and mind toward others. People with a warm personality are likable, empathetic, and get invited to parties. Everyone is attracted to their charisma, playfulness, intuition, and expressions of compassion.

HEART NETWORK

The physical and mental correlations for the Heart Network include: Heart and small intestine, blood vessels, tongue, blood, perspiration, intuition, and compassion. The function of this group controls blood flow, temperature regulation, and empathic virtues—all having some degree of warmth and movement. The Heart nourishes the HeartMind with blood and qi in the MDT where we use it to communicate with other sentient beings. Then with further development through qigong and meditation the Spirit will migrate to the UDT. Although expanding the HeartMind to develop the Spirit is a natural process for all of us, it seems to come most readily to the "Fire type."

The Fire type person will tend to have a slender physique with graceful hands, long arms and legs, and a lean neck. Their long fingers taper toward the tips, the skin is thin and often reveals the underlying blood vessels, and their complexion tends to be light and pinkish. Fire personalities crave excitement, drama, intimacy, and movement. They like to be understood and always want to know what you are thinking. Mystery and hidden meaning appeal to their sharp intuition and sense that there is more to life than meets the eye. They have a profound desire to be intimate with all living things. The Fire type easily resonates with the Summer Qigong path that leads to spiritual awakening.

Our life depends on fire; it comes from the Heart Qi. Fire from the Heart gives joyful vitality to our lives. A deficiency of Fire will show signs like fatigue, low blood pressure, edema of the legs, lethargy, chills, or a deep internal feeling of coldness; we withdraw and become less talkative, preferring to be alone. Excessive Fire symptoms could present as mania, insomnia, anxiety, neurological tremors and spasticity, profuse sweating, high blood pressure, and, of course, cardiac arrest.

Everyone benefits from doing Summer Qigong. The Fire type will be energetically balanced and happily on the path to awakening. Those who have a deficiency of Fire should emphasize the active qigong exercises in the program. And those with too much fire will benefit by paying particular attention to the meditation practice.

HEARTMIND

Our capacity for expressing positive human values comes from the *xin*, often translated as HeartMind, a compound word implying that the Heart's emotional knowledge combines with the mind's rational thinking to give us a uniquely human perception of the world. When our actions are appropriate to the situation, considerate of others, and done with good intentions, the HeartMind is vibrant and lovingly engaged with the world.

The HeartMind must be carefully nurtured if we want to follow the path of spiritual awakening.

Chinese medicine tells us that the HeartMind develops from the joining of Liver Blood and Heart Qi in the MDT. We deliberately cultivated that energy field with Spring Qigong practice. Now in this season we should continue to elevate the vitalized blood and enriched qi to achieve higher realms of consciousness where we live beyond the restraints of egocentric thoughts and behavior, thus experiencing the full flowering of human fellowship and divine nourishment.

When we enjoy loving relationships, perform altruistic deeds, and wish the best for others, the HeartMind has established intimate personal and social relationships that promote the greater good of our communities. In addition to interpersonal communications, we can nurture the HeartMind in a way that feeds our hunger for higher love. This advanced development takes place in the MDT through qigong and meditation practice—the HeartMind is transformed into Spirit, which then ascends through the *Taiji Axis* to reside in the UDT. With further dedicated practice, the Spirit comes awake and we dwell in a world of serene selflessness.

How to Practice

All qigong practice sessions should begin with "Awakening the Qi" (see page 118) and should end with "Sealing the Qi" (see page 132). This opening and closing will integrate body and mind with the energy centers and channels of qi circulation. Awakening the Qi serves as an energetic warm-up by stirring the LDT with your hands, calling to the upper dan with your fingertips, and warming the Kidneys with massage. Sealing the Qi concludes the practice by bringing the energy back to the LDT; in this way you do not lose the wonderful health benefits just gained.

When you finish a qigong movement, do the "Cleansing Breath": Bring your feet together, stand with your arms relaxed down, your spine comfortably erect, and your eyes gazing softly into the distance. Take a deep inhalation, and then audibly and completely exhale through your mouth. Stand quietly for a few moments, intentionally point your fingers toward earth and feel the qi circulating through your body. Too often people will fidget around after doing a qigong exercise or rush into the next movement; this dissipates the energy that was just cultivated. The Cleansing Breath allows the qi to continue moving along the intended course, thus enhancing energy flow and mental equanimity. Most importantly, it brings you back to earth so that you remain rooted to this source of energy throughout the practice routine. It only takes a brief time to do, so do not neglect this important centering exercise.

Most styles of qigong have three aspects to every exercise: body movement, mental intention, and rhythmic breathing. These three factors have shifting proportions depending on the season. Summer Qigong highlights mental intention. While doing these exercises, always be aware of the HeartMind, knowing that it is the source of love and goodwill; at the same time be conscious of the Yang Qi radiating outward to make contact with heaven and earth. Let your mind be as spacious as the clear blue sky. Put some effort (gong) into Summer Qigong and reap the rewards of the Heart Qi awakening your consciousness to the common desires of all human beings to feel safe, to be accepted, and to be healthy.

SUMMER QIGONG

> In the three months of summer, it is important to be happy and
> easygoing and not hold grudges, so that the energy can flow freely
> and communicate between the external and the internal.
>
> (*The Yellow Emperor's Classic of Medicine*)

This season's practice centers on the culmination of Supreme Yang Qi development: forming warm interpersonal relationships and then creating wholehearted connections with the Dao. As the wellspring of limitless energy, the Dao enfolds the earth and the universe in a benevolent embrace; its basic principle proclaims that every human being has the core virtue of essential goodness. Our destiny is to fully realize basic goodness, to express it, and to help others know it as well. The presence of kindness, generosity, and love signify spiritual awakening. The process begins with cultivating Heart Qi.

Awakening the Qi

Warm the Dan Tian

Use your right palm to rub 36 times clockwise around your navel. Then replace your right palm with your left and rub 36 times counterclockwise.

Beat the Heavenly Drum

Cover your ears with the heels of your hands. Then tap with the fingertips on your occipital bone for about 10 seconds.

Massage the Kidneys

Form loose fists with your hands, then massage up and down over your lower back 36 times.

Do Awakening the Qi only once.

Northern Star

Start by standing with your feet together and your hands at your sides. Then shift your weight onto your right leg.

Inhale as you lift your left arm out in front and then overhead (Figure 7.2). Your left palm faces forward, your fingers spread like the rays of a star. Think of standing tall with a vertical connection between earth and heaven.

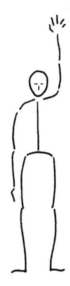

Figure 7.2: Northern Star

Exhale slowly through your mouth as you lift your right arm and left leg out and up in a diagonal line (Figure 7.3). Do this in front of a mirror while training—it will help you align your diagonal arm and leg.

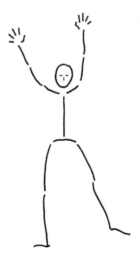

Figure 7.3: Northern Star

At the end of exhaling return to the starting position with your hands at your sides and feet together.

Inhale as you shift your weight to your left leg and raise your right arm out and up (Figure 7.4).

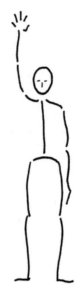

Figure 7.4: Northern Star

Exhale as you lift your left arm and your right leg out to form a diagonal line (Figure 7.5). Both your palms face forward, with your fingers spread. Your chest is lifted, and your gaze is straight ahead.

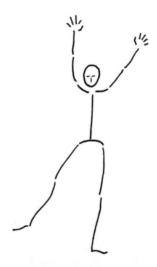

Figure 7.5: Northern Star

At the end of exhaling return to the starting position.

Inhale and shift your weight to your right leg, raise your left arm and repeat the movement.

Do eight repetitions.

Visualize that your "solar plexus" (just below the sternum) is a pivotal point where vertical and diagonal lines of energy from earth and heaven are flowing through your body.

Mixing Yin and Yang

Stand with your feet wide apart and your hands at your sides. Bend forward at the waist, then squat down until your hands touch the floor and cross your wrists with your palms up (Figure 7.6). It does not matter which wrist is on top.

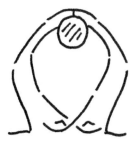

Figure 7.6: Mixing Yin and Yang

Inhale slowly as you stand up; as you do so, your crossed hands turn in toward your chest, then they roll down and forward with your wrists still crossed (Figure 7.7). This is the "mixing" action of energy through the LDT. The crossed wrists with the arms close to the body is a very yin posture. Inhaling is a yin activity.

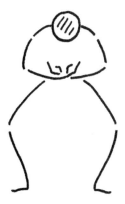

Figure 7.7: Mixing Yin and Yang

Continue inhaling until your crossed wrists are overhead, and your knees are straight (Figure 7.8). This is the end of the inhalation.

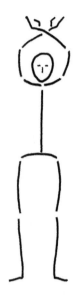

Figure 7.8: Mixing Yin and Yang

Exhale slowly through your mouth as you uncross your wrists, spread your arms laterally, circle your arms down with your palms facing laterally, and bend your knees (Figure 7.9). The spread of the arms with palms facing outward with exhalation is a very yang expression.

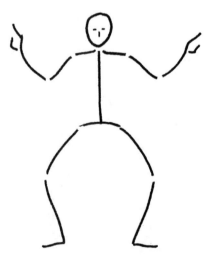

Figure 7.9: Mixing Yin and Yang

Inhale gently as you straighten your knees and lift your palms up to your solar plexus (Figure 7.10).

This is a rather short inhalation.

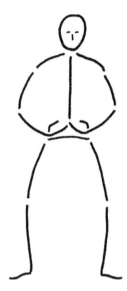

Figure 7.10: Mixing Yin and Yang

Exhale as you bend forward at the waist, with your knees almost straight to get a stretch in your hamstrings and lower back (Figure 7.11). Your wrists are not crossed.

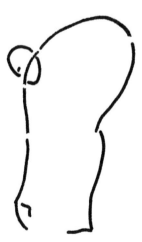

Figure 7.11: Mixing Yin and Yang

Finish the exhalation as you squat down and cross your wrists with your palms up (Figure 7.12). Either hand is on top.

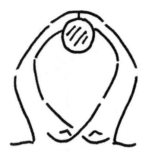

Figure 7.12: Mixing Yin and Yang

Inhale and repeat the movement. Do eight repetitions.

Visualize that you are lifting yin energy out of the earth, mixing it through the LDT, and transforming it into the yang energy of heaven.

Waiting at the Temple Gate

Stand with your feet wide apart and your hands at your sides.

Inhale slowly into the LDT.

Exhale through your mouth as you bend over from the waist (Figure 7.13). Your knees are straight but not locked. Relax with your head and hands down toward the floor; feel a nice stretch in your hamstrings.

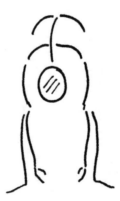

Figure 7.13: Waiting at the Temple Gate

At the end of your exhalation, give the floor/earth a sharp tap with your fingertips, like flicking water off the fingers. There should be an audible sound from the tapping. Think of this as calling forth energy from the earth.

Now squat down with your elbows touching inside your knees (Figure 7.14). Your arms extend to the sides, your palms facing forward in an open posture.

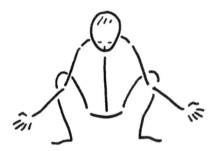

Figure 7.14: Waiting at the Temple Gate

Inhale slowly as you stand up with your arms moving outward and upward in a large circle (think of this as gathering energy from the environment). Continue inhaling as your knees straighten (Figure 7.15).

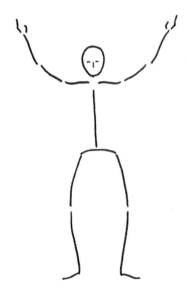

Figure 7.15: Waiting at the Temple Gate

Finish the inhalation when your hands meet overhead in a prayer posture (Figure 7.16).

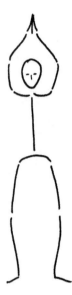

Figure 7.16: Waiting at the Temple Gate

Exhale very slowly through your mouth and bring your hands down the midline to the level of your heart (Figure 7.17). Then sharply and audibly give a final exhalation as you quickly bend your knees so that you are in a semi-squat. Your hands remain in prayer position at the MDT.

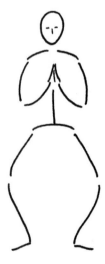

Figure 7.17: Waiting at the Temple Gate

Inhale as you stand up and lower your hands to your sides. Stand comfortably erect.

Exhale as you bend over and repeat the movement. Do this three times. At the end of the third repetition hold the semi-squat praying hands position (Figure 7.17) and take three slow breaths. While doing this, let the phrase "What does it mean to be waiting at the temple gate?" drift through your mind. Lightly contemplate "waiting," "gate," and "temple." You may or may not have an answer. It doesn't matter; you are simply planting a seed of spirituality into your consciousness.

Heart Qigong

This qigong practice will calm the *HeartMind* and elevate the Spirit. Done in three steps with a nice even rhythm, it equally uses the three aspects of qigong: body movement, breathing, and mental intention. This qigong exercise is an all-time favorite with many of my students as it smoothly activates the three *dan tians* with a pleasant pumping action of open/close and up/down movements guided by the breath and concentration. Many people feel this internal energy moving after only a little practice. The combined mental intention, regulated breathing and body motion create a strong connection between earth and heaven by raising the qi up through the *Taiji Axis*. An important factor that makes Heart Qigong a premier exercise for the Fire Phase is the use of *Shanzhong* as an energetic focal point during the practice. This energy gate controls the qi flow as it moves through the middle *dan tian. Shanzhong* is located on the midline of the chest, eight finger-widths below the clavicles. It is a master point often used in acupuncture and qigong for opening the chest to relieve stagnation of qi, relaxing the Heart and reducing anxiety, conveying energy and information through the *Taiji Axis*, and nurturing kindness and communication.

Begin by standing with your feet about shoulder-width apart, and your hands at your sides. Slightly bend your knees. Mentally make contact with the "Bubbling Well" acupuncture point on the soles of your feet just behind the toes. Bring your hands to the LDT with the palms up and middle fingertips almost touching (Figure 7.18).

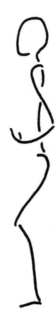

Figure 7.18: Heart Qigong

Inhale and slowly lift your hands up to your chest as your palms turn toward *Shanzhong*, and straighten your knees (Figure 7.19). Finish inhaling.

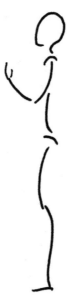

Figure 7.19: Heart Qigong

Visualize gathering qi from the earth, and bringing it up to the MDT.

Exhale through your mouth and turn your palms away from your body; push your hands outward and away in an arc (Figure 7.20). Bend your knees. Finish exhaling, with your arms extended laterally and your palms facing out.

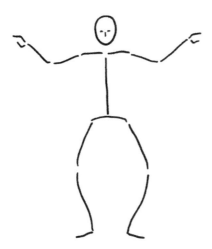

Figure 7.20: Heart Qigong

Visualize exhaling any toxins or stress from your chest.

Inhale, bend your elbows as if you were encircling a ball (Figure 7.21), and bring your hands back to *Shanzhong* as your knees straighten.

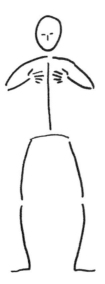

Figure 7.21: Heart Qigong

Think of bringing fresh qi into your Heart.

Exhale, bend your knees, and keep your palms facing *Shanzhong* as you finish exhaling (Figure 7.22).

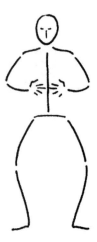

Figure 7.22: Heart Qigong

Visualize healing qi sinking into your Heart.

Inhale slowly, and let your elbows down so that your forearms are vertical, your wrists are touching, and your fingers are up with your forearms parallel as your knees straighten. Your hands form a "flower" under your chin (Figure 7.23).

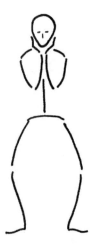

Figure 7.23: Heart Qigong

Finish inhaling when your hands are straight up above your head (Figure 7.24).

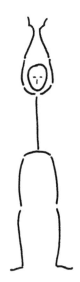

Figure 7.24: Heart Qigong

Visualize lifting your Spirit to the heavens.

Exhale as your arms open widely and circle downward, your knees bend and your hands descend to the level of the LDT with the palms up (Figure 7.25), as in the beginning position.

Visualize returning your Spirit to earth.

Do eight repititions.

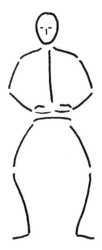

Figure 7.25: Heart Qigong

Sealing the Qi

Whole Body Tapping

Use your palms to tap over each arm, your trunk, outer legs, inner legs, abdomen, lower back (use your fists on your back). Do this three times.

Arms Horizontal

Put your arms straight out to the sides, with your fingers pointing up, for one breath.

Heaven and Earth

Inhale and lift your hands laterally and then overhead, with the palms pointing to heaven. Rise up on your toes and hold your breath for a few seconds. Slowly exhale, lower your heels, and with your palms facing the earth, lower your hands to the LDT.

Seal

Cover the LDT with the palm of your right hand. Place the palm of your left hand over your right hand with the thumb tucked under your right hand. Stand quietly for three breaths.

Do Sealing the Qi only once.

SUMMER MEDITATION
The Colors of Health

Each of the major yin organs—Heart, Lung, Liver, Spleen, and Kidneys—has a healthy affinity for a specific color—red, white, green, yellow, blue—because each of these colors has a frequency on the visible light spectrum that resonates with the electromagnetic energy in each organ. Resonance, whether of color or sound, amplifies the innate healing power within the organs.

The Colors of Health meditation utilizes intense visualization to project color into one organ at a time. In this meditation, you intensely visualize appealing colors that you have actually seen. For example, a fresh red berry, new white snow, spring green grass, rising yellow sun, deep blue ocean. The energy of that light—captured when it entered the brain through your eyes—stays within your mind and can be activated with intention. This inner retained energy can then be sent into the organs with the Colors of Health meditation.

Another part of this meditation employs powerful affirmative feelings that go hand in hand with the attitude of "kindness." When we sincerely express the emotions of kindness and goodwill there is a cascade of positive neuropeptides released into the blood by the central nervous system. When these chemical compounds reach the organs they stimulate a "parasympathetic response" from the autonomic nervous system that has a widespread calming and healing influence on all organ networks. This generalized effect becomes more specific when we project the appropriate color into the proper organ; the combination of vivid color and positive emotions has tremendous healing potential for many illnesses. The two techniques—visualizing color and extending kindness—meld into a beautifully relaxing and vibrant journey through your interior landscape.

Begin the meditation by comfortably sitting or lying on your back. Take a few slow deep breaths. Now look inward with a gentle smile. If you actually form a small genuine smile, like smiling to yourself in the mirror, it will naturally bring forth kindness. Just express a nice pleasant smile, as if you are looking at a favorite pet.

Take your time with each organ. Deeply visualize its color; use a shade and intensity that appeals to you. Extend feelings of gratitude to that organ for all that it has done to keep you alive every minute of your life. Whether the organ is healthy or unwell, project a sense of kindness and goodwill as if it were a close friend or loved one. Give each organ at least two or three minutes of your loving attention. Then remain seated for another few minutes with no particular thoughts in your mind. Feel a colorful, calm spaciousness throughout your chest and abdominal areas.

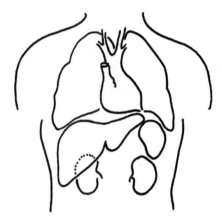

Figure 7.26: Colors of Health

Sunflower Meditation

The sunflower represents the blooming of the Spirit in the Heart. You can cultivate this awakening by using the energy of your own smile. When you smile inwardly (as you did in the Colors of Health meditation) it evokes the feeling of loving kindness for yourself, and ultimately, for all others. This powerfully simple meditation can instill a state of deep contentment, centeredness, and being at peace with the way things are. The sunflower symbolizes the *HeartMind*—the emotional intelligence that makes us fully human. The HeartMind enables us to use consciousness, empathy, and compassion to effect warm and amiable interpersonal socialization.

Sit comfortably with your eyes closed, and breathe softly through your nose. Become aware of the ebb and flow of your breath through your body. Relax. Feel the rise and fall of your lower abdomen and ribs. Breathe like this for a little while and let your mind settle down.

Calmly pay attention to your breath. Let all of the ten thousand thoughts that are trying to grab your attention float by, like clouds across the sky. Be mindful of your breath coming in and going out. Don't follow the thoughts—just let them go, and come back to the breath.

As distracting thoughts dissolve away, you begin to look inward at the area around your Heart. *Imagine a small sunflower in the center of your chest* (Figure 7.27). Look at it. Smile to it. Just smile. Just look. Breathe normally, comfortably, and in a relaxed manner.

Think of *bathing the flower with your smile*—as if you were looking at a loved one, with gentleness and a feeling of sending goodwill to your beloved.

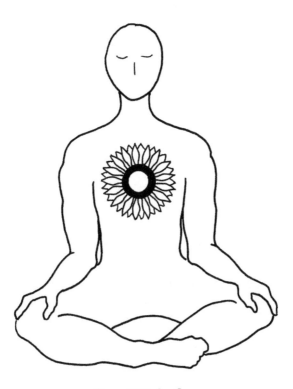

Figure 7.27: Sunflower

See the colors of the sunflower. Notice the richness and depth of color. See the details in the petals, the wonderful variations of bright yellow and deep reds and a soft green. You are looking, breathing, smiling, giving the flower your loving attention.

As you meditate on this flower, *see how it slowly grows in size.* It gets larger until it fills your chest. There is a feeling of relaxing so that your chest can open. The warm colors brighten your Spirit. Just gaze at the flower and behold its beauty.

Feel that your abiding, benevolent smile to the sunflower is the energy that gives it life and vitality. *When you are smiling to the sunflower you are connected to HeartMind the source of kindness and inner tranquility.* Feel this gentle power of your smile soak into your entire body, like water into dry soil. Let yourself relax into the energy of your own loving smile. Simply breathe.

And now see that as you gaze at it *the sunflower slowly becomes smaller with each exhalation.* The image becomes smaller and smaller until it disappears.

The enduring love of your smile is still there, but not seen. What remains is the feeling of openness in your chest, peace in your mind, and love in your Heart. Continue sitting with this sense of inner calm and contentment for a few more minutes.

HEART, HEARTMIND, AND SPIRIT

Your life depends on your heart maintaining an absolutely essential rhythm 24 hours a day, 365 days a year. Take a moment right now, relax, breathe deeply, and be thankful for what this amazing muscle does—without much thought from you—every minute of your life. Of all the internal organs, the Heart makes the strongest connection between your physical body and emotional life. Yang Qi powers the pump to establish a rhythmic pulse that continuously alternates between moving the blood and resting. Blood functions as the most yin substance of the Heart; it carries nutrients, hormones, and antibodies to keep you healthy and in touch with the world. Yin Qi of the Heart nurtures not only your objective existence but also your subjective sense of love, contentment, and social rapport. If the yang and yin aspects of the Heart are thriving and interacting in mutual support, they create the totality of Heart Qi.

If the Heart Qi is weak, we suffer. On the emotional level we become disinterested, inarticulate, and joyless around our friends and associates. We lack the spark of life and become less warm blooded and more "reptilian." Deficient Heart Qi on the physiological level may exhibit conditions such as cardiac insufficiency, atherosclerosis, or orthostatic hypotension. On a higher plane, a lack of Heart Qi prevents us from attaining the spiritual satisfaction of awakening to our true nature, of realizing our fundamental goodness as the essence of our being. The full potential of being human never comes to fruition. A robust Heart Qi expresses the vitality of positive emotional fire. Its energy feels like a burst of loud laughter—startling but also compelling. It ignites a compassionate connection with humanity and all earthly souls, while at the same time it seeks a dimension of awareness that connects with celestial spiritual energy.

Humans are animals. We have basic needs, like all life forms, for food and shelter. And like all animals, we have a physical body that must be fed from the bounty of the earth. But humans exist as unique sentient beings. Our bipedal bodies have extraordinary capabilities and our complex minds have superlative cognition, but more than that, we have a special awareness that can make contact with the divine realm of being—human consciousness harbors both mind and Spirit. We know how the machinations of the mind can cause global destruction and how rational analysis has created techno-scientific wonders. We also have seen how the human Spirit creates transcendental music and art, builds breathtaking temples, rescues other beings from hardship, and—ultimately—yearns for contact with sacred worlds.

Because a healthy body depends on good nutrition, *Qigong Through the Seasons* presents unique recommendations for foods and herbs that have special value at each season. These dietary guidelines help you absorb and utilize the vital energy of nature; they also assist mental function and spiritual development. However, our desire for spiritual fulfillment requires a different kind of nourishment not found in food. The sustenance for feeding the Spirit comes from the combined practice of qigong and meditation.

This Spirit, called "*Shen*" in Chinese, is unique to humans because it is the source of intelligent compassion, a trait that makes us different from other animals. This Spirit evolves from the cultivation of the HeartMind in the MDT through qigong and meditation. With dedicated practice, the *Shen* flourishes and migrates to the UDT where further transformation returns the Spirit to the great Void. Our Spirit contains the whole range of consciousness and emotions, as well as the human quest for a meaningful life.

When this Spirit makes contact with the Dao, the primordial source of life, we reach a level of intimacy with all things that surpasses our earthbound bodies. Keep in mind that "universe" means "one song," which tells us that everything on earth and in the heavens is interdependent. All spiritual traditions acknowledge this sense of universal oneness as the greatest expression of the human Spirit.

Each of us has a unique experience of the Spirit world. Although a natural part of being human, spirituality is difficult to describe with words; thus it not often discussed. But trust the process of qigong and meditation. Spiritual awakening is as real as being in love. It may happen only once, or be a progression of happenings. It may seem to last forever, or be gone with the next breath. On the ultimate plane of consciousness, Spirit exists more so than your body. Have faith in the process. Be diligent in practice. Enjoy this mysterious journey, which is fulfilling beyond words, and well worth the effort.

THE FIVE SPIRITS

The term "*Shen*" has multiple uses. I have been discussing the *Shen* that relates to the Heart, summer, and the Fire Phase. However, the Chinese consider that there are five different types of *Shen*, or Spirits, embodied in a human being. Each Spirit is responsible for a particular virtue (Kaptchuk 2000) that comprises an identifiable personality. This concept of five incarnate Spirits has allowed Chinese doctors to treat those nonphysical aspects of a person through the organ networks. Each Spirit is attached to a particular organ and can be influenced by qigong, acupuncture, herbs, or meditation directed to the associated organ. These Spirits are independent of any religious belief; they are inherent capabilities and tendencies that fill out the human condition.

1. The *Yi* implies intention, thought, and decision making. As you have seen, we use intention quite often in our practice when we mentally direct or visualize energy movement. In that context it functions as an indispensable part of qigong. But *Yi* has a broader definition when considered to be the virtue of sincerity, honesty, and authenticity. Our *Yi* helps us to make decisions and see potential consequences of our actions in regard to other people's needs and situations. Part rational analysis and part emotional candor, the *Yi* prompts us to do the right thing for the greater good of others in our families and communities. The *Yi* is associated with the Spleen. If the Spleen becomes sluggish and weak the *Yi* declines into worry, lassitude, confusion, and possible depression.

2. The *Hun*, often translated as "non-corporeal soul," carries with it that deeply Confucian virtue of *ren* or human kindness. While the *Yi* allows us to think about, analyze, and formulate a plan of action in regard to others' predicaments, the *Hun* compels us to make an immediate emotional connection to those in need, to recognize their suffering and to act on their behalf with heartfelt compassion. It is said that the *Hun* survives the death of the body in the sense that it is the memory

people have of a deceased person's good deeds and the benevolence that they exhibited during their lifetime. In both life and death, the *Hun* is a person's "good name." On a personal level, the *Hun* relates to the Liver, and if that organ network becomes dysfunctional, the *Hun* becomes disturbed with manifestations of anger, rage, jealousy, revenge, and resentment.

3.   The *Po* lives with the Lungs; if breathing stops, the *Po* disintegrates. Sometimes referred to as the "animal soul," the *Po* can be considered a corporeal soul in that it is very much attached, almost literally, to the body. Spontaneous action, passion, and unthinking reactivity define one aspect of the *Po* that operates as an instantaneous presence in moment-to-moment life. The virtue of the *Po* is its sense of "preciousness" (*bao*)—that ability to "capture the perfection and completeness of a single moment," (Kaptchuk 2000 p.65). It exhibits a bodily reaction to the beauty of singular acts of pure humanity: profound awe of great art, complete integration with divine power, and total appreciation of this treasured human life. If the *Po*—or its organ correspondent, the Lungs—becomes disrupted, a person never has a sense of completion or things coming to their proper resolution; this is most troublesome, giving rise to the emotion of grief.

4.   The *Zhi* ("jur") is the Will that resides in the Kidneys. It has two definite aspects. The first, the Yang Will, is readily recognized as "willpower" or the capacity of volition, determination, and dedication to a closely held personal principle of conduct. When we apply effort (the "gong" in "qigong") toward achieving a high level of physical skill, scholastic recognition, or artistic expression, we are operating with the Yang Will. The other side, the Yin Will, is an elusive concept but is akin to having a sense of destiny about the course of our life, of knowing that life's unfolding is deeply beneficial to our spiritual awakening, or on the other hand, that our current trajectory is leading us toward disappointment, despair, or great unhappiness. The Yin Will exerts a gradual righting of the ship if it has drifted off course in the sea of a lifetime. Both the Yang Will and the Yin Will have the virtue of wisdom. This is a profound trust that our decisions and actions will eventually have positive outcomes because the bedrock of our being is basic goodness.

And though this inherent morality seems too often concealed to be known, it is wisdom that allows us to trust in and search for the great mysteries of human life on this planet. A weakness in the Kidneys' Yin or Yang may lead to a feeling of incompetence, aimlessness, and a serious dissatisfaction with our present life.

5. The fifth Spirit, *Shen*, resides in the Heart and aligns closely with the concept of HeartMind in that it has to do with interpersonal communications. If the Heart is dysfunctional, we become aloof or even antisocial; we will be unable to attach a value to anything beyond our bodies. Our *Shen* enables us to establish an unconscious but very real connection by looking a person in the eye as we speak, genuinely listening to what they are saying, choosing words that offer comfort or understanding, and generally "clicking" with another person. The social virtue of this Heart Spirit is the Confucian concept of *li*—propriety, ceremony, ritual, familial allegiance—all aspects of behavior that leads to communal cohesion. Another virtue of the *Shen* is strictly personal. It is that human yearning to make contact with divine reality in order to feel, to be, completely human—to experience an ineffable state of knowing that body, mind, and Spirit exist as the ultimate manifestation of energy. When defining the indivisibility of the body and the mind, an esteemed contemporary scholar says, "spirit and body are nothing but two different states of condensation and aggregation of Qi," (Maciocia 2009, p.4). His statement applies to all five *Shen* in that they each represent a specific synthesis of emotional, cognitive, and psychic energy centered on a particular organ network. The *Shen* of the Heart, at its highest level of development, allows us to understand beyond thinking that we belong to a community that surpasses culture; we live in a collective region of the universe where every moment contains compassion for all things.

So what is the relationship between the Five Spirits and qigong or mediation? How can you use this information in your practice? The sages of Chinese medicine have identified special virtues that form the nonphysical part of human life and give it added value beyond mere animal existence. As your practice develops and you become comfortable with tranquility and inner focus, you should take time to contemplate the meaning of these virtues. Each of them is connected to one of the Five Phases, so you may want to give special attention to cultivating the virtue that pertains to the current season. However, each trait exists at all times. The *Yi* relates to the Spleen and the Earth Phase; and because that phase is eternally present, the virtues of honesty, sincerity and helpfulness should be a constant in your life. The *Hun* takes helpfulness and adds kindness to give you the admirable traits of empathy and compassion for the plight of other people. The *Po* allows you to demonstrate a full appreciation for daily life and the fruits of artistic expression. The *Zhi* functions like a bridge between being engaged in society and moving further along the path of your personal destiny. Finally, the *Shen* leads you to experience spiritual awakening and the full revelation of your humanity. These profound components of your personality have been given names so that you can identify them and know when they are present in your life. They are the best parts of who you are, so give them the attention they deserve.

SUGGESTIONS FOR SUMMER PRACTICE

Some Daoist traditions hold that we should practice four times a day when the 24-hour yin–yang cycle has transition periods: dawn/Rising Yang, noon/Supreme Yang, dusk/Gathering Yin, midnight/Ultimate Yin. Doing seasonal qigong practice during the time that coincides with yin–yang circulation can enhance the effects. The period from 11:00 am to 1:00 pm would be ideal for most people to do Summer Qigong practice, especially those who have a deficiency of fire. However, the Yang Qi is very strong at high noon, and individuals who are already too yang because of excessive fire should not practice at this time; it is better for them to do the practice in the morning when the qi is naturally rising and will gently augment the practice. Morning practice is best for almost everyone.

There are several ways to combine qigong exercises and meditations into a practice routine. My daily work schedule varies so that sometimes I only have 10–15 minutes to practice in the morning, whereas on other days I can devote time to a longer session of an hour or more. There are many ways to divide the exercises and meditation into groups. Here are some suggestions for putting what you have learned into different qigong/meditation sets that have a particular emphasis:

1. Awakening the Qi; Northern Star; Heart Qigong; Sealing the Qi; Colors of Health Meditation. *Cultivates ascendant Qi.*

2. Awakening the Qi; Waiting at the Temple Gate; Heart Qigong; Sealing the Qi; Sunflower Meditation. *Cultivates Heart Qi.*

3. Awakening the Qi; Northern Star; Mixing Yin and Yang; Waiting at Temple Gate; Heart Qigong; Sealing the Qi; Colors of Health Meditation or Sunflower Meditation. *Complete cultivation of Summer Qi.*

Consider the intention of each exercise as you make your sets for practice; experiment with various groupings; notice how certain groups are internally or externally biased. You should approach and perform your practice with a sense of play, curiosity, and openness. Although traditionally practiced in the morning, the important issue is to make practice fit in with the rest of your schedule. Don't let it become a conflict, but don't neglect it either.

FOOD, FLAVORS, AND HERBS FOR SUMMER

The *bitter* flavor is closely identified with the Fire Phase and the Heart. Bitter foods and herbs will cool heat, clear stagnation of the blood, and correct damp conditions that can cause too much mucus, edema, and skin eruptions. Bitter will benefit those individuals who are too watery, lethargic, overweight, and slow, as well as those who are too hot, aggressive, or scattered.

We in the West tend to think that the bitter flavor is less satisfying than sweets, salt, and fats. It doesn't spike our blood sugar, tickle our tongue, or give us that sense of comfortable satiety. But when we stop and think about the common foods we eat and drink we see that bitter is all around us.

Coffee and tea are tied for second after water as the most widely consumed drinks in the world; they stand as perfect examples of the bitter flavor. Also bitter: romaine lettuce, bok choy, radicchio, and celery. Many foods are a combination of bitter and other flavors: bitter and sweet (asparagus, most lettuce, papaya, quinoa); bitter and pungent (citrus peel, radish, scallion, turnip, white pepper); bitter and sour (vinegar). A healthy diet will include some degree of bitter foods based on personal taste and availability.

SINGLE HERBS FOR CARDIOVASCULAR HEALTH

While we should increase our consumption of flowering, leafy fruits and vegetables in summer, we should also eat those herbs and foods that have been shown to benefit the Heart and the expression of *Shen*, regardless of the season. Single herbs as well as combinations of herbs in specific formulas can promote healthy cardiovascular function and emotional balance.

Garlic (Allium sativum) reigns as one of the world's most respected medicinal plants for the Heart. More than 1100 scientific articles and over 250 research studies have shown that this odorous plant can effectively lower elevated cholesterol and triglyceride levels. Just one clove of garlic a day can reduce the tendency of blood to form life-threatening clots by 50–80 percent. (Those people taking blood-thinning medication should seek their physician's advice before consuming garlic.) For those who prefer to avoid the smell of regular garlic consumption, it may be taken in capsules or tablets. You will get the highest concentrations of allium and other beneficial sulfur compounds by chopping or pressing freshly peeled garlic cloves.

Hawthorn (Crataegus laevigata) has a favorable effect on the cardiovascular system. When used long term, the leaves may help with palpitations, hypertension, angina, and atherosclerosis. As a mild sedative, it helps with anxiety and stress. Hawthorn berries can reduce symptoms of food stagnation, such as gas, belching, and abdominal distention. In powder form, take one to two capsules, two to three times daily. As a tincture, mix two to three dropperfuls in water and drink two to three times daily. If you were to take only one medicinal herb for various problems in the cardiovascular system, hawthorn would be a great choice (used, of course, only in consultation with a licensed health care practitioner).

A HERBAL FORMULA TO CALM THE SPIRIT

Supreme Yang Qi marks the extreme limit of yang energy in nature; all living beings are filled to capacity with energy that should bring joy and exuberance to their activities. For most people, the fullness of Heart Qi manifests as warm, relaxed, and convivial relationships—but not for everyone. A person who has a deficiency of qi can have a difficult time in summer. The season's hyperactivity can be overwhelming to those without sufficient Heart Qi to receive, control, and absorb the Yang Qi from nature. This constitutional deficit predisposes the person to an overriding apprehensiveness that often makes them anxious, easily frightened, giddy, and forgetful. They can also have heart palpitations and may exhibit neurotic behavior. Incessant or inappropriate laughter shows up as a distinct symptom of deficient Heart Qi occurring in summer; it signals a lack of personal qi that cannot control the environmental yang energy. These people often display hyperactivity and glee that hides an exhausted and disquieted Spirit; they are running on empty and cannot keep up with the speed of Supreme Yang Qi.

"Settle the Emotions Pill" has been used for generations as a basic herbal formula for nourishing Heart Qi and calming the *Shen*. The classic recipe has only four ingredients: ginseng (*ren Shen*), poria (*fu ling*), acorus (*chang pu*) and senega root (*yuan zhi*). Ginseng and poria augment the qi in general, while acorus and senega root calm the Spirit and settle the emotions. For patients who have a weak or very sensitive constitution, codonopsis can be used instead of ginseng for milder qi tonification that will not overstimulate them. "Settle the Emotions" can treat a wide range of psychological problems including obsessive–compulsive disorder and anxiety neurosis. Always seek professional help if you feel that deficient Heart Qi could be a problem for you. There are many variations on this valuable formula that a qualified herbalist can recommend. You should always consult a knowledgable herbalist before using medicinal herbs.

RECIPES FOR SUMMER

Salads, in all their magnificent diversity, are the superior foods for the summer season. They are fresh and full of the yang energy typically found in ripening fruits and vegetables. Interestingly, the foods that grow during the Fire Phase are replete with water. Eating them may help mitigate the effects of heat, both externally and internally.

For thousands of years, the field of Daoist dietetics has suggested that we should eat foods of many colors. Research from modern food science supports this ancient prescription for healthy eating. The Produce for Better Health Foundation[1] has compiled a list of the phytochemicals and benefits that are found in fruits and vegetables of different hues. As you read this information, think of the foods that have these colors:

- *Blue/Purple*: Anthocyanins and phenolics that lower the risk for some cancers, benefit the urinary tract, may improve memory, and promote healthy aging.

- *Green*: Lutein, indoles, and many other chemicals that lower the risks for breast, prostate, and lung cancer, promote eye health, strengthen bones and teeth, and boost immunity.

- *White/Tan/Brown*: Allicin, genistein, and phytosterols benefit the heart by slowing cholesterol absorption and lower the risk of breast, lung, and other cancers.

- *Yellow/Orange*: Bioflavonoids, carotenoids, and limonoids for better eye and heart health; they also boost immunity.

- *Red*: Anthocyanins, catechins, cholorgenic acid, and lycopene for better memory and heart health; they also protect the urinary tract, boost the immune response, and lower the risk of many cancers.

---

1   The Produce for Better Health Foundation's website can be found at www.pbhfoundation.org.

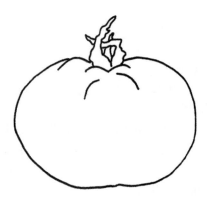

Green Salads

For a perfect Heart tonic salad use any combination of romaine lettuce, bok choy, celery, and radicchio. The bok choy should be "baby boks" for the tender leaves. Slice the leaves rather than tear them. Slice the stalks as you would the celery. A little radicchio adds tang and color to this green salad. Use your favorite tangy dressing.

Baked Fruit

(Serves 4)

Raw fruit salads are, of course, very popular in summer. But for a different use of these gifts from nature, try this simply delicious recipe.

2 tbsp pure maple syrup

2 tsp lemon juice

1 tsp pure vanilla extract

Pinch of salt

5 cups sliced soft fruits (e.g., peaches, plums, apricots, pineapple, and mangoes) or 5 cups harder sliced fruits (e.g., apples and pears)

Preheat the oven to 400ºF (250ºC/Gasmark 6).

Mix the maple syrup, lemon juice, vanilla extract, and salt together in a bowl. Add the fruit and mix well. Put the mixture in a 9-inch square baking pan.

Bake, stirring once or twice, for 15–20 minutes for the soft fruits, or 35–40 minutes for the harder ones.

Serve plain, or with yogurt or granola.

A healthy diet for the Heart and the qi of summer will include daily salads of varying ingredients but with an emphasis on bitter greens and vegetables such as romaine, bok choy, radicchio, and celery. Green tea complements these salads very well. Eat quinoa as a bitter-flavored source of protein. Use a lot of garlic for its lipid-lowering effects and for its delicious flavor. Take hawthorn as a tea or in capsules for a mild cardiovascular tonic. If, after reading the above information, you think that you have symptoms of Heart Qi insufficiency, you should consult a licensed practitioner of herbal medicine. The right combination of food and herbs can help you harmonize with and enjoy the energy of Supreme Yang Qi in the Fire Phase.

CHAPTER 8

AUTUMN

METAL PHASE

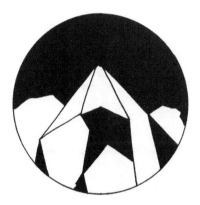

Autumn invites contemplation of your present and future. You should decide what you want to keep in your life and what to discard. The waning autumn season emboldens you to let go of what has been depleted and to prepare for winter and self-preservation. At this autumnal time of year many people feel a mild melancholia, a need to yawn, a desire to curl up in the slanting sun and nap the afternoon away. But this sense of slowing down also prods us with the feeling that there is work to be done. You must take time to separate the wheat from the chaff, to finish those outdoor chores, and then to get your house—body and mind—in order.

But let us enjoy these glorious autumnal days while they last. The gentle sun, the just-right temperatures, the splendid colors that are like gems of perfection—each adds to a sense of deep contentment. Like leaves floating down from the trees, every moment makes a special journey through a fleeting phase of time. At this season the energy of nature descends toward earth, the sap returns to the roots. Plants contract on the stalk and shunt their energy into vital seeds for regeneration; animals put on thick coats and layers of fat for protection from the coming cold. Autumn is a season of beautiful fulfillment and transient climax that overlays a serious preparation for self-preservation.

Jin ("gin"), the character for metal (see Figure 8.1), has three components: a sloping roof indicating an overlying cover, three horizontal lines connected vertically, indicating layers within the earth, and two short energetic lines at the bottom implying nuggets of metal deep in the earth (Hicks, Hicks, and Mole 2004, p.130). *Jin* represents a precious treasure, small in size but large in value, laying buried underground.

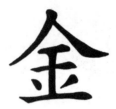

Figure 8.1: Metal character

People throughout the world, in all ages, have sought to craft treasures of the earth—diamond, jade, gold, silver—into objects that would beautify their bodies and adorn their domiciles. Metals have always had a universal appeal for their domestic functionality, visual charm, and military advantage. One of the first cultures to mine and refine ore, the ancient Chinese developed metallurgy to a degree unattained by the rest of the world for centuries. From iron, copper, and zinc they developed utensils, tools, and weapons that advanced their societies beyond pre-civilized impoverishment. What's more, Chinese alchemists and physicians sought further transformation of base metals into gold and internal elixirs in their quests for methods to improve health and, hopefully, attain immortality.

In the practice of *Qigong Through the Seasons*, the Metal Phase relates to riches hidden within your body and mind. The Three Treasures of humanity are *Jing*, *Qi*, and *Shen*—the elemental forces that shape human life (see Chapter 1). Each Treasure receives special attention during each of the four seasons; the Metal Phase focuses on the Descending Qi of autumn. After the climax and scattering of summer's Supreme Yang Qi, nature retrieves the essential qi from the world and brings it downward for storage and gestation, whether in a tree's roots, seeds on the ground, or in the LDT. Within the ceaseless recycling of yin and yang, the period when the qi descends—autumn—is known as the season of Gathering Yin. The Metal Phase empowers us to cut through illusions of identity, to eliminate mental distractions, and rein in the hyperactivity of summer. As days grow shorter and nights get colder, you should make decisions regarding the direction of your life—are you happy, healthy, and content with the way things are? Or do you have questions and doubts about relationships, material things, jobs, locations, careers—does there seem to be a sense that things could, and should, be better? Are there obstacles that must be overcome on the path of your destiny? The practice of Autumn Qigong can help you address and answer critically important questions about your life.

LUNG NETWORK

The elements of the Lung Network address issues of defense, separation, and rhythm. Lungs, the large intestine, nose, mucous membranes, and skin all exist to maintain boundaries between the outside environment and our body's interior in order to acquire beneficial energy, while protecting us from noxious external influences and eliminating internal waste products. Emotionally, the Lung Network relates to grief, loss, and detachment. The dominant theme for the Metal Phase revolves around decision making, sensitivity to external influences, and self-made principles.

People exhibiting traits of the Metal Phase will have a compact, trim body with small, but developed, musculature and a defined bone structure. They give the impression of a well-cared for physique that doesn't take up much room. The "metal type" likes precision, rationality, and ceremonial beauty; they take pleasure in contemplating the poignant metaphor of falling leaves, noticing the sharp edge of an autumn breeze, and making preparations for the coming cold weather. A tendency toward asthma, bronchitis, and chest colds plagues them in autumn; their inherently dry skin may easily develop rashes or eczema. The Metal type does very well with bookkeeping, analytical projects, formal designing, and other activities that require discrimination, synthesis, and decorum. However, they can become indifferent, aloof, and withdrawn in domestic relationships, or dictatorial and overly critical in professional encounters. Generally autumn is their favorite season and, if they can avoid respiratory problems, they feel right at home in the Gathering Yin time of year. Autumn Qigong appeals to the Metal type because of its emphasis on measured breathing, graceful movements, and healthy Lungs.

THE SOURCE OF QI

Breathing stands out as our quintessential rhythmic interaction with the world: Lungs function as a permeable interface between each of us and everything else. The Lungs are yin organs that receive air from the outside world, extract its healthy components and send them downward to the LDT to combine with the nutrients of food. That fusion of air's vitality and food's energy produces our greatest quantity of qi. In ancient times, the word "qi" primarily had the meaning of "vital breath" emphasizing that our indispensable energy comes from breathing. One Chinese character for qi pictures steam rising from a cooking vessel, indicating the transformation of food into active energy. In the practice of internal alchemy, a subset of qigong, the qi vessel represents our LDT, which functions like a stove for heating and converting food into qi. Air and food are equally important for a healthy lifestyle; that's why qigong exercises and a diet based on seasonal energetics are staples in the practice of *Qigong Through the Seasons*.

When we take in Heaven Qi—air—we become inspired with a vitality that circulates through the body, keeping us alive and healthy. The ability to take in a complete natural breath equals our potential to be inspired by the full impact of everything life offers. Too often we breathe only from our upper chest, which limits the amount of oxygen going into our bloodstream. We should breathe like we did as infants, from the belly, so that the Lungs fill to capacity with oxygen, hydrogen, nitrogen, and other nutrients from the air. Then, at the completion of the breath cycle, we exhale the unused portion of air to be recycled into the atmosphere.

Astonishingly, the lungs eliminate 70 percent of the body's waste products. This makes exhalation a hugely significant detoxifying activity. We must completely exhale so that the respiratory system can flush out toxins and debris; only then can we receive a full complement of fresh air on the next inhalation. Stress, fear, anger, and doubt are the main emotional states that interfere with a healthy exhalation. Many people subconsciously don't let go of the breath—

they feel like they must hold on to that last bit of air, otherwise they may expire. The ability to completely let go of the breath often relates to issues of trust and relaxation. The correct practice of qigong creates mental tranquility and thus will profoundly enhance healthy breathing by relaxing the Lungs and allowing them to function freely.

The Lungs also act to spread the *Wei Qi* ('way chee') or Defensive Qi that protects us from external pathogens. As a special type of energy, the Defensive Qi resides on the skin and mucous membranes, where it acts as an agent of self-defense. The skin, the largest organ of the body, functions as our most obvious encounter with the external world; it relays sensations from the outer world to the brain, protects us from threatening organisms and injurious accidents, and also eliminates waste products through perspiration. The large intestine is the yang counterpoint to the Lungs; it also serves to protect us by separating the good from the bad. The colon recycles water and minerals from the intestinal mass to form a compact waste product for elimination. Problems with this organ are often related to the physical and/or mental inability to relax and "let go."

You should respectfully consider the Lungs, skin, and large intestine as your Secretaries of Defense. They are responsible for protecting the boundaries—both physical and mental—that separate you from the rest of the world. These three organ systems, as integral aspects of the Metal Phase, play a central role in health care during autumn.

Four Phases of Breathing

In daily life, we usually take for granted or totally ignore that which keeps us alive. The most important thing we do from moment to moment is breathing. So profoundly simple and yet utterly imperative, breathing ensures life. If we can't breathe, nothing else matters. And many people don't breathe well. The importance of the breath has been recognized by all cultures as a vital link between body and mind, the external and the internal. Breath's rhythmic pattern keeps us inwardly together in all respects. Outwardly, the unceasing flow of air through ourselves links us to the natural world and to all of its resources:

Chuang Tzu, the seminal Daoist philosopher, distinguishes the deeply grounded presence of a true sage from that of ordinary people by highlighting the central importance of breathing:

The True Man breathes with his heels,

his breath comes from deep inside;

the mass of men breathe with their throats,

they gasp out their words as though retching.

(Watson 1996, p.74)

Inhalation is an active process with a short pause at the end. Exhalation is a passive process that ends with a longer pause. Many qigong masters consider that moment of neither inhaling nor exhaling to be a rest stop on the highway of life—the Daoists call it a "moment of immortality." It is a timeless state when we may be totally at peace, when the border between our self and the world dissolves, when we stop becoming and just be. Let's explore this process of breathing.

Sit or lie down comfortably on your back and relax. Just let your breath do what it will. Don't try to control anything. Just watch for a while. Then slowly begin to rest your attention on your exhalation. Feel that gentle contraction of your body as the breath goes out. Notice that momentary pause just after exhaling. Let yourself relax there. Don't hurry. Trust your body. When it needs to take another breath in, it will. As you surrender to this restful pause you may find that it lengthens on its own. The wisdom of the body seeks this still point where it can completely relax without thought or movement: a moment of immortality!

Now, begin to rest your attention on your inhalation. Feel how the body inflates as the muscular diagram gently pushes the ribcage outward. This wonderfully subtle expansion brings in fresh air to vitalize your life. Again notice that pause at the end of inhaling. It is naturally shorter than the pause after exhalation but nevertheless still there and noticeable.

Relax. Enjoy the comfort of natural breathing. Linger at the rest stops on the highway of life.

HOW TO PRACTICE

All qigong practice sessions should begin with "Awakening the Qi" (see page 156) and should end with "Sealing the Qi" (see page 169). This opening and closing will integrate body and mind with the energy centers and channels of qi circulation. Awakening the Qi serves as an energetic warm-up by stirring the LDT with your hands, calling to the upper dan with your fingertips, and warming the Kidneys with massage. Sealing the Qi concludes the practice by bringing the energy back to the LDT; in this way you do not lose the wonderful health benefits just gained.

When you finish a qigong movement, do the "Cleansing Breath." Bring your feet together, stand with your arms relaxed down, your spine comfortably erect, and your eyes gazing softly into the distance. Take a deep inhalation, and then audibly and completely exhale through your mouth. Stand quietly for a few moments, intentionally point your fingers toward earth and feel the qi circulating through your body. Too often people will fidget around after doing a qigong exercise or rush into the next movement; this dissipates the energy that was just cultivated. The Cleansing Breath allows the qi to continue moving along the intended course, thus enhancing energy flow and mental equanimity. Most importantly, it brings you back to earth so that you remain rooted to this source of energy throughout the practice routine. It only takes a brief time to do, so do not neglect this important centering exercise.

Most styles of qigong have three aspects to every exercise: body movement, mental intention, and rhythmic breathing. These three factors have shifting proportions depending on the season. Autumn Qigong accentuates breathing. You will learn how to breathe correctly and how to use the breath cycle to generate copious amounts of good healthy Qi. You will experience the exquisite timelessness of the embryonic breath as well as the dynamic interaction of breathing and body movement as a crane and a tiger. Be sure to come back to the Cleansing Breath after each qigong movement.

AUTUMN QIGONG

> Autumn is the changing point when the yang phase turns into the yin phase.
> This is the time to gather one's spirit and energy, be more focused,
> and not allow desires to run wild. Keep the lung energy full, clean and quiet.
>
> (*The Yellow Emperor's Classic of Medicine*)

Qigong practice for the Metal Phase begins with two exercises for spinal flexibility and loosening the ribcage. "Circling Sparrows" creates greater lateral flexion of the ribs and spine while also improving range of motion in the shoulders. "Breathing from the Kidneys and the Lungs" is one of my all-time favorite qigong exercises. It works externally on the spine, the anchor of our skeleton, and internally on the Kidneys and Lungs—the only organs that come in pairs—which facilitates bilateral polarity of qi flow through the trunk. The practice then progresses into selections from the famous "Five Animal Frolics," crane and tiger. These seriously playful exercises enhance the relatively yin-crane and yang-tiger qi of the Metal Phase. "White Healing Mist" combines body movement, regulated breathing, and mental intention into an elegant internal qigong exercise that is remarkably helpful for healing lung disorders; it reigns as the foremost practice for Autumn Qigong.

Awakening the Qi

Warm the Dan Tian

Use your right palm to rub 36 times clockwise around your navel. Then replace your right palm with your left and rub 36 times counterclockwise.

Beat the Heavenly Drum

Cover your ears with the heels of your hands. Then tap with the fingertips on your occipital bone for about ten seconds.

Massage the Kidneys

Form loose fists with your hands, then massage up and down over your lower back 36 times.

Do Awakening the Qi only once.

Circling Sparrows

Begin by standing with feet close together and hands at your sides.

Inhale as you bring your right hand overhead, and put your left hand at the level of your belly (Figure 8.2). Your palms are facing each other and aligned on a vertical axis; your elbows are slightly bent.

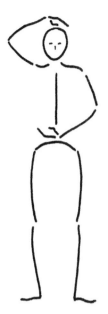

Figure 8.2: Circling Sparrows

Exhale and bend to the left, letting your arms and hands extend a little (Figure 8.3). Think of your hands as two birds playing in the air, making smooth circular motions.

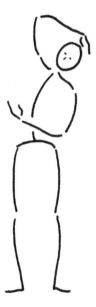

Figure 8.3 Circling Sparrows

Inhale as you come back to the center, then change hand positions so that your left hand is above your head and your right hand is at the level of your belly. *Exhale* as you bend to the right and circle the sparrows.

Visualize qi flowing through the arms and hands.

Do 12 repetitions.

Breathing from the Kidneys and the Lungs

Begin by letting your breath out as you bend forward, with your knees slightly unlocked, and hang there comfortably (Figure 8.4). Feel a stretch in your lower back.

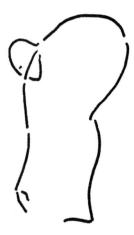

Figure 8.4: Breathing from the Kidneys and the Lungs

Inhale, remain bent over and feel your lower back expand. Your Kidneys are tucked up under your lower two ribs. Think of inhaling qi into your Kidneys.

Exhale as you straighten up and put your palms on your lower back over the Kidney area.

Extend slightly backward, look upward, stay in that position and *inhale* from your chest (Figure 8.5). Feel your chest expand. Think of inhaling qi into your Lungs.

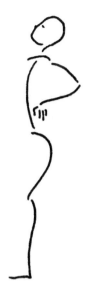

Figure 8.5: Breathing from the Kidneys and the Lungs

Exhale, bend forward, and repeat the movement.

Visualize your lower back and chest expanding with fresh qi.

Do eight repetitions.

Crane Frolic

The qi cultivating exercise known as the Crane Frolic is part of the famous and highly revered "*Five Animal Frolics*" developed by Hua Tu sometime around 150 CE. According to Professor Ken Cohen, a luminary in the world of qigong practice and research, "The Five Animal Frolics is the most ancient qigong system still practiced today" (Cohen 1997, p.199).

The Five Animal Frolics involve short sets of graceful movements based on the traits of crane, bear, monkey, deer, and tiger; they form a comprehensive exercise system comprising all three major types of qigong: medical, martial, and spiritual. In the 1970s there was a great resurgence of interest in the Five Animal Frolics due to Gou Lin, an actress from Beijing who recovered from cancer by practicing them. She successfully led the movement to include qigong therapy in hospitals, and it has since developed into an integrated aspect of health care in most of China's hospitals, clinics, and community centers.

The Crane Frolic is especially good for nurturing the qualities of lightness, balance, endurance, and stillness. It benefits the Heart and Lungs by increasing the circulation of qi in the upper body; it brings more blood to the muscles and sinews of the shoulder girdle structures. It builds strength in the legs and is ideal for developing better balance. I have had students who could not stand on one leg for ten seconds before doing the Crane Frolic, but gained significant leg strength and could balance on one leg for more than a minute after only six weeks of practice.

After doing the six Crane exercises people often have a feeling of greater tone and openness of the upper back, shoulders, and chest, as well as a calmly focused mind and sturdy legs. Many cultures look to the crane as a symbol of longevity, achieved through graceful body movements and a keen, penetrating mind.

Note: Do the entire Crane Frolic slowly and smoothly without stopping. Do not do the Cleansing Breath in-between the six exercises.

Basic Crane Stance

Stand with your feet close together, heels almost touching, and toes pointing outward. Your knees are unlocked. Your hands are down at the sides of your legs. Breathing is through the nose unless otherwise indicated.

Crane Breathing

Place you hands in front of LDT, with the palms up and the middle fingers almost touching (Figure 8.6).

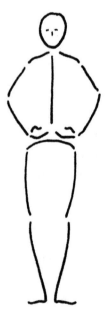

Figure 8.6: Crane Breathing

Inhale, and lift your hands up to your chest. Your palms face skyward, your shoulders stay down (Figure 8.7). Think of your elbows like a crane beginning to open its wings as they move out and flex.

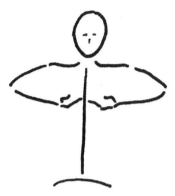

Figure 8.7: Crane Breathing

Exhale as your hands descend to the LDT, with palms up as in Figure 8.6.
Do eight repetitions.

Crane's Beak

From the end of Crane Breathing go straight into Crane's Beak. Lift your arms laterally and upward until they are horizontal at shoulder level, your palms facing the earth (Figure 8.8).

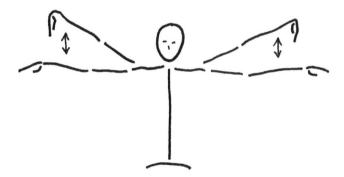

Figure 8.8: Crane's Beak

Inhale, and form the Crane's Beak by bringing all five fingertips together and pointing downward. Lift the arms/beak higher until your hands are just above head level.

Exhale while you open your hands, straighten your wrists, and lower your arms until they are again horizontal at shoulder level with open palms facing the earth.

Do eight repetitions.

Crane Flaps Wings

From the end of Crane's Beak, continue exhaling, and lower your hands down to hip level. Keep your palms parallel to the earth (Figure 8.9).

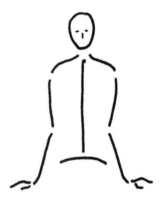

Figure 8.9: Crane Flaps Wings

Inhale and lift your arms/hands up to shoulder level. (Figure 8.10) Keep your arms horizontal and your palms level with the earth.

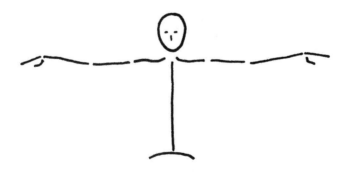

Figure 8.10: Crane Flaps Wings

Exhale and your lower hands to hip level. Bend your wrists to keep your palms parallel to the earth, as in Figure 8.10.

Do eight repetitions.

Crane Squats and Turns Wings

Inhale, squat down comfortably, lift your heels off the floor, turn your palms skyward and lift your arms up to shoulder level as in Figure 8.11.

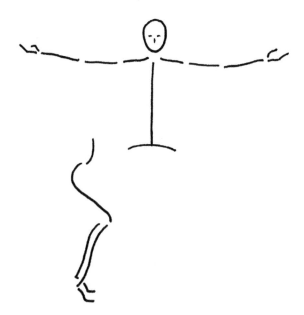

Figure 8.11: Crane Squats and Turns Wings

Exhale through your mouth, lower your heels to the floor, stand up, turn your palms toward the earth, and lower your arms to hip level as in Figure 8.9.

Do eight repetitions.

Crane Stands on One Leg

From the end of Crane Squats and Turns Wings, continue exhaling through your mouth, and squat down. Lower your hands to the floor and cross your wrists (Figure 8.12).

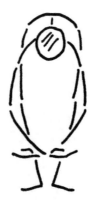

Figure 8.12: Crane Stands on One Leg

Inhale, stand up, shift your weight to your right leg, and lift your crossed hands overhead, with the palms facing toward the rear. Raise your left leg off the floor, and bring your knee up until your thigh is parallel to the floor (Figure 8.13). Your ankle is relaxed with your toes pointing downward.

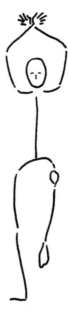

Figure 8.13: Crane Stands on One Leg

Continue inhaling as your wrists uncross and your arms circle out and down to shoulder level with your palms facing the floor (Figure 8.14). Your left knee remains raised, with your thigh parallel to the floor.

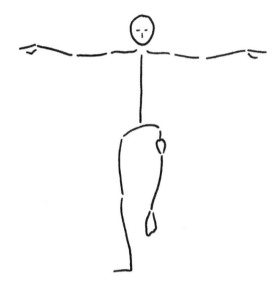

Figure 8.14: Crane Stands on One Leg

Exhale, lower your foot to the floor, squat down, and lower your hands to the floor as in Figure 8.12. Completely exhale through your mouth.

Do eight repetitions, alternating left and right.

Crane Spreads Wings

Stand with your feet close together, heels almost touching, and toes pointing outward. Your knees are unlocked, and your hands are at your sides (Figure 8.15). This is the Basic Crane Stance.

Inhale, shift your weight to your right leg, step forward and slightly to the left with your left foot, letting your toes gently touch the ground. Keep your arms straight and your elbows near your sides. Roll your shoulders backward, and turn your palms outward. Keep your weight on your rear leg.

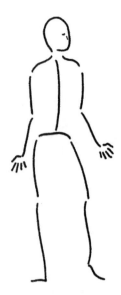

Figure 8.15: Crane Spreads Wings

Exhale and bring your left foot back beside your right foot. Your body turns straight forward. Roll shoulders forward, and turn your arms until your hands are touching back to back (Figure 8.16). Shift your weight to your left leg and continue.

Do eight repetitions, alternating left and right.

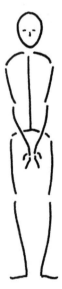

Figure 8.16: Crane Spreads Wings

White Healing Mist

This graceful *neigong* (internal qigong) exercise fills the Lungs with fresh qi while cleansing them of turbid qi. The intent of the mind uses detailed imagery of pure and impure qi. The movement of the hands leads the qi into and out of each Lung. The "white healing mist" can be any personal image that conveys a sense of purity, freshness, tranquillity, and healing. The "toxins" can be not only respiratory debris but also cloudy, unhealthy thoughts. As the interface between our internal and external worlds, the Lungs command our self-defense system. When doing this practice, you may want to identify those healthy and unhealthy aspects of your life. Then nurture the good with the white mist, and purge the bad along with the toxins. Do this exercise slowly with focused concentration on one Lung at a time. The unilateral emphasis is unusual since most qigong exercises are done for both Lungs simultaneously, but that special concentration on one Lung at a time increases the concentration of qi, which makes this a very powerful healing exercise. You can do this for the common chest cold and for all serious diseases of the Lungs.

Begin with your feet close together, and your hands crossed and touching your chest over the Lungs (Figure 8.17). Your right hand is over your left Lung and your left hand is over your right Lung.

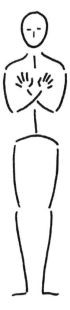

Figure 8.17: White Healing Mist

Take a slow, relaxed breath and *think of your Lungs there under your hands*. Make a mental connection between your hands and your Lungs.

Step to the side with your left foot. Your hands are still crossed on your chest (Figure 8.18).

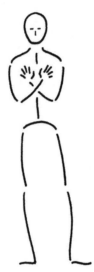

Figure 8.18: White Healing Mist

Inhale and shift your weight onto your left leg so that your left Lung is aligned with your left knee. At the same time, open your arms and slowly swing your hands forward and then laterally out until your arms are extended to the sides with your fingers up and your palms facing away from your body (Figure 8.19). Your left knee is bent, and your right knee is straight.

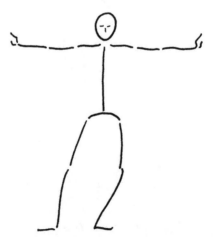

Figure 8.19: White Healing Mist

Think of inhaling a white healing mist into your left Lung only.

Exhale, step back to center with your left foot, and straighten your knees. Return your hands to your chest, and cross them so that your right hand is touching your chest over your left Lung. Your left hand touches your chest over your right Lung.

Think of exhaling grey smoky toxins from your left Lung only. Although both hands are touching your chest, your focused intention goes to your left Lung only.

Repeat for your right Lung by stepping to the right, etc.

Do eight repetitions, alternating left and right.

Sealing the Qi

Whole Body Tapping

Use your palms to tap over each arm, your trunk, outer legs, inner legs, abdomen, and lower back (use your fists on your back). Do this three times.

Arms Horizontal

Put your arms straight out to the sides, with your fingers pointing up, for one breath.

Heaven and Earth

Inhale and lift your hands laterally and then overhead, with the palms pointing to heaven. Rise up on your toes and hold your breath for a few seconds. Slowly exhale, lower your heels, and with palms facing the earth lower your hands to the LDT.

Seal

Cover the LDT with the palm of your right hand. Place the palm of your left hand over your right hand with the thumb tucked under your right hand. Stand quietly for three breaths.

Do Sealing the Qi only once.

AUTUMN MEDITATION

The following three meditation practices will bring clear awareness to your mind, fresh qi to your body, and deep serenity to your Spirit whenever you do them.

Medicine Man Breathing

Qigong exercises place a great emphasis on intentional breathing. The diaphragm, as the major muscle of respiration, establishes the fundamental yin–yang rhythm of the body. When it contracts, air is drawn into the Lungs; when it relaxes, air is expelled. This rhythmic movement of the muscular diaphragm controls more than the inflation and deflation of the Lungs; it also pumps lymphatic fluid through every tissue of the body. The lymph system gathers up cellular waste products, runs them through filters, and then returns the clean fluid as plasma into the bloodstream. Modern science has, through microscopic observations, described this process of internal cleansing in detail. However, pre-modern people have practiced intuitive methods of interior purification for thousands of years by purposefully directing the breath, and therefore the Qi, through the major entry and exit portals of the meridian system—the palms of the hands and the soles of the feet.

Healers from many different cultures recognize the importance of the breath for good health. These men and women use breathing techniques to purify the body, focus the mind, and open the Spirit. This has been happening for as long as people have been on the earth. As more technological cultures come to realize that their own medicines are not entirely adequate to help with the needs of the whole person, they begin using some of these timeless breathing methods to evolve a true holistic medicine.

Fools Crow was a famous medicine man of the Teton Sioux, revered for curing sickness and for his exceptional spiritual life. This man devoted every moment of his existence to nurturing the physical and spiritual aspects of his people. His life is documented by Thomas Mails in *Fools Crow: Wisdom and Power* (Council Oaks Books, 1995). To prepare himself for healing sessions, Fools Crow would do a simple yet profound technique that I call "Medicine Man Breathing," which I have adapted and changed from Fool Crow's original practice to incorporate specific breathing methods, acupuncture points, and qigong principals. He would often do this while lying on the top of a grassy hill with nothing but the clear blue sky around him. Fools Crow has given us an exquisite gift for self-healing; we should practice it with a sense of gratitude.

Lie on your back with your arms comfortably by your sides and your palms facing the sky. Relax your entire body and mind.

Inhale slowly through your nose and at the same time think of breathing in through the *laogong* points in the palms of your hands. Gently open your hands by extending the fingers. Think of the fresh air coming into your Lungs through your nose and, at the same time, up your arms from your palms. Thus, fresh qi surges into your Lungs from two sources: your nose and your hands.

Exhale slowly through your mouth as you lead the qi down through the center of your body, washing all the internal organs, to the LDT where the Descending Qi divides and goes down the center of both legs to the bottom of your feet—like a warm wind of fresh energy. Finish exhaling out the *Bubbling Well* points on the soles of your feet just behind the base of the toes. It helps to slightly extend the toes to open up the exit points. Think of getting rid of debris, toxins, and tension at the bottom of your feet.

Repeat this purifying exercise as many times as you wish. Try it while lying in warm grass with the sounds of nature all around and the limitless sky above.

Breath Counting—A perfect practice for the Metal Phase

This intriguing practice is especially appropriate for autumn as we are focused on nurturing the Lung Qi during the Metal Phase. Mindfulness and awareness the cornerstones of meditation will carry your mind along the breath toward equanimity and good health. However you use it, the breath cycle will always be available to assist in the discovery of your true nature. The Descending Yin Qi of the Metal Phase concentrates your powers of discrimination, judgment, and decision making so that you can carefully examine the contents of your life and make changes that benefit your health.

Breath Counting meditation gives you the opportunity to clear your mind and contemplate your destiny.

Begin by sitting upright on a cushion or chair. Hold your spine comfortably erect with hands resting on thighs with palms down, or in your lap with palms up and one hand on top of the other. If you sit on a meditation cushion (*zafu*), your knees should be bent and legs crossed in one of the following positions: both feet on the floor one in front of the other (natural lotus position), or one foot resting on the lower leg of the other (half lotus), or both feet resting on the lower part of the opposite leg (full lotus). If sitting on a chair, your feet should be flat on the floor; the chair seat should also be flat to facilitate uprightness. You may also choose to sit on a specially designed bench (*seiza*) where the lower legs tuck beneath the seat. A timer can be helpful to set an allotted period to practice: 10, 20, 30 or more minutes are good options.

Relax, and just become aware of your breath coming in and going out. Don't try to control the cycles, just watch them. The breath cycle has four stages: inhalation, pause, exhalation, and pause. Again, put your attention on the breath cycles for a minute or two; become aware of the four parts of breathing. Notice how the pause after exhalation extends out longer than the pause after inhalation. Daoists call that lingering pause after exhaling "a moment of immortality."

Now, begin to *silently count your exhalations from one to ten*. Notice what happens. Many thoughts will flicker through your mind. The goal is to not become attached to those thoughts; don't dwell on them. You simply keep letting go of the thoughts and constantly bringing your mind back to the count. If you forget the count just go back to one. Relax. Almost everyone will lose track of the count at times because a thought carried their mind away. It commonly happens. The most important issue is that you do not get caught up in self-criticism—no judgments—just come back to the breath. If you do reach the count of ten, return to one and continue counting the exhalations up to ten again, and again. Eventually you will become peaceful and undisturbed by the thoughts that move through your mind like clouds across the sky. Then, after the chosen time has expired, let go of counting the breath and simply rest in tranquility. Let that moment of immortality linger a little longer.

Embryonic Breathing

After Breath Counting you may want to refine your awareness with Embryonic Breathing. This practice creates such a subtle, effortless, and calm presence that you become almost motionless. It connects you to the vastness of space and eternity—as if you returned to the womb to become immortal. Embryonic Breathing can lead you to a timeless level of awareness as expressed by a modern qigong master: "When an adult practices Embryonic Breathing, he or she feels a return to the womb of the universe, nurtured by the primordial qi. The breath is so slow, easy and slight that it seems to have stopped" (Cohen 1997, p.125). Similar to the "moment of immortality" at the end of exhalation, Embryonic Breathing liberates the Spirit from the bonds of time.

Entire books have been written on Embryonic Breathing. The most comprehensive is *Qigong Meditation: Embryonic Breathing* by Yang Jwing-Ming (YMAA Publications, 2003). In the first 322 pages, Dr. Yang explores the entire spectrum of qigong research, from ancient documents to modern studies. The actual practice of Embryonic Breathing makes up the last 24 pages. The depth of historical research and the author's commentary illustrate the high regard Embryonic Breathing has in the canon of qigong sacred texts.

Do the meditation in a seated position; if lying down, you have the real possibility of going to sleep and this is not the purpose of Embryonic Breathing. However, you may go to bed after this practice and enjoy a restful and restorative night.

For the first few minutes, mindfully cultivate the five qualities of Daoist breathing: *slow*—as in slow down; *long*—an extended pause after exhalation; *fine*—breathe through the nose; *even*—make your inhalation and exhalation the same length; *deep*—down to the bones.

After a while, let go of any thoughts about the quality of your respiration. Simply become quiet. Enter stillness. Be there as long as you want.

SUGGESTIONS FOR AUTUMN PRACTICE

The following components make up the Autumn Qigong practice. You can use them to build your personal two-part program of qigong and meditation. Explore each of them, try them on, and see how they fit. Have fun but be serious. The summer parties have come to an end; now the clear air of autumn sharpens your perception about what really matters and what does not. Conduct your days with an eye toward identifying the detritus of unhealthy habits and situations. Look for those positive aspects of your personal relationships, career, and lifestyle that nurture the Three Treasures—essence, energy, Spirit—and do everything you can to enhance their presence in your life.

The ideal practice is to do everything listed under "Qigong." This takes about ten minutes. Add any of the "breath meditations." Breath Counting and Embryonic Breathing flow together nicely. Medicine Man Breathing is a fine way to finish the qigong practice. You could do qigong and meditation during the same session, or you could do them at different times of the same day, or you could do qigong one day and meditation the next. However, be sure to do at least one of the breath meditations with any *short* practice. Make a commitment to do at least some part of the practice every day.

A short practice could take many forms, including the three below:

1. Awakening the Qi; Circling Sparrows; Breathing from the Kidneys and the Lungs; White Healing Mist; Sealing the Qi. (6–8 minutes.)

2. Awakening the Qi; Crane Frolic; White Healing Mist; Sealing the Qi. (8–9 minutes.)

3. Awakening the Qi; Circling Sparrows; Breathing from the Kidneys and the Lungs; Sealing the Qi. (7–8 minutes.)

The amount of health benefits you get from a qigong/meditation practice directly relates to how often you practice. Regularity of practice is more important than the length of a session. Each person will obtain unique benefits, but some of the first and most common are as follows: a feeling of being at ease in your body and calm in your mind; feeling that all body parts are united and harmonious; having a more optimistic view of life; projecting a sense of confidence and tranquillity; having more energy throughout the day; and sleeping better at night. For these reasons, daily practice has great rewards.

The Lungs can suffer from prolonged grief. Everyone at some point will have a shattering experience of deep loss. I once had a 14-year-old patient who was brought to me by her mother because the child had severe asthma unrelated to allergies. She had gone through various drug treatments with little success, so now they wanted to try Chinese medicine. My examination revealed a definite deficiency in Lung Qi and Heart Yang Qi. The child's father had died suddenly two years previously—her asthma began six months later. We did an initial course of acupuncture and herbs for two weeks; the wheezing was somewhat reduced and she seemed a little less anxious. But I wasn't satisfied with the results. At the next visit I began a gentle inquiry about the loss of her father. The mother became so distraught that she had to leave the treatment room. The child seemed to open up and said that she couldn't stop thinking about him: "Why did he die? There's a big hole in my life." Grief is a normal emotion that should be fully expressed and eventually brought to closure. This child had no closure. I taught her the White Healing Mist exercise; she liked the idea of doing something active, and practiced the movement daily. We continued with acupuncture once a week, and within a month she and her mother had noticed a remarkable improvement in the frequency and intensity of the asthma attacks. Healing occurs on many levels.

FOOD, FLAVORS, AND HERBS FOR AUTUMN

The seasonal circulation of our internal energy can be enhanced by eating specific types of food that correspond to the direction of qi circulation in the natural world. In spring the energy moves up; in summer the energy moves out; in autumn the energy moves down; and in winter the energy moves inward to the core of the body. The physical traits and growing habits of foods support this movement within us. Green, sprouting foods are best for spring. Flowers and leaves that grow outward are best for summer. *Downward growing vegetables are best for autumn.* Dense, concentrated grains, seeds, and nuts are best for winter.

Eating from a local garden will maintain the connection between your diet and the four directions.

For autumn we should look to carrots, potatoes, onions, turnips, beets, and other earth-dwelling foods as the major ingredients in our diet. These foods are the primary carriers of yin energy. Our next choice should be those foods that ripen on the surface of the ground, such as squashes and pumpkins. A diet that combines foods below and just above ground level is ideal for autumn. Also, any other foods ripening at this time of year are appropriate. The yang energy of apples, plums, and pears will nicely balance the yin-dominant foods mentioned above. Finally, you should round out your diet by picking those items from the grain, meat, dairy, and vegetable groups that are easy to digest.

Sour correlates to the season of Gathering Yin because it has a cooling, contracting, gathering, and astringent action. It tends to consolidate the qi and move it downward. Sour has a great energetic affinity for autumn because it gathers together much of the energy in our body that was dissipated in the Fire Phase of summer. Everyone can benefit from eating foods with the sour flavor during the time of Descending Qi. The taste of sourness comes from the acidic quality of foods; citric acid and tannic acid are common sources. Most people would do well to eat more sour foods such as lemon, lime, pickles, rose hips, hawthorn berry, sauerkraut, and vinegar.

Pungent, a yang flavor, ventilates the Lungs. Because it has a dispersive, drying, and warming action, it helps prevent congestion in the respiratory system. During autumn the Lungs will accumulate qi as a result of the universal movement of energy throughout nature from outside to inside and from above to below. Pungent foods will protect against excessive qi in the Lungs that may cause bronchitis, asthma, or a chest cold.

The Lungs are sensitive to the balance of moisture and dryness; they should be moist—not too dry and not too wet. Excessive servings of pungent and spicy foods will tend to dry the Lungs, so the therapeutic use of such foods should be only for conditions of too much mucus, as in sinus infections or a cold. However, it is wise to eat small amounts of pungent foods for Lung tonification on a regular basis during autumn. Some of the most useful include cayenne, garlic, ginger, cinnamon, onion, red and green peppers, spearmint, fennel, dill, basil, and nutmeg.

RECIPES FOR AUTUMN

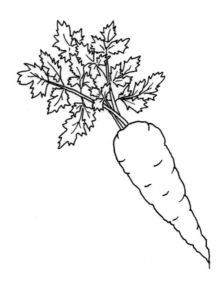

Russian Cabbage Borscht

(Serves 4–5)

This beautiful soup makes the perfect autumn meal. The wonderful ground-dwelling beets, potatoes, and carrots are combined with the yin–yang flavors for the Metal Phase: vinegar (yin), and both dill and caraway (yang). Enjoy this soup with wholegrain bread and butter.

2 tbsp butter	1 large carrot, sliced
1 cup thinly sliced beets	3 cups chopped cabbage
1½ cups thinly sliced potatoes	black pepper to taste
4 cups stock or water	¼ tsp dried dill
1½ cups chopped onion	1 tbsp + 1 tsp cider vinegar
1 scant tsp caraway seeds	1 tbsp + 1 tsp honey
2 tsp salt	1 cup tomato purée
1 stalk celery, chopped	

Place the beets, potatoes, and stock in a saucepan and cook until everything is tender. Drain the vegetables and reserve the stock.

Begin cooking the onions in the butter in a large pot. Add the caraway seeds and salt. Cook until the onions are translucent, then add the celery, carrots, and cabbage. Add the reserved stock. Cover and cook slowly until all the vegetables are tender.

Add the beets, potatoes, and all the other ingredients to the vegetables in the large pot. Cover and simmer for at least 30 minutes. Add seasoning to taste.

If you wish, serve topped with sour cream.

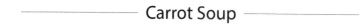

Carrot Soup

(Serves 4–6)

The simplicity of this dish belies the deep flavor that develops from the alchemical mixing of the carrot, orange, cardamom, cayenne, and butter. A superb soup for nurturing Autumn Qi.

4 lbs (2 kg) carrots, cut into 1 inch rounds	8 tbsp butter
2½ cups chicken stock	½ cup fresh orange juice
2½ tsp ground cardamom	1½ tsp salt
¼ tsp cayenne pepper	

Place the carrots in a large pan, cover with water, and bring to a boil. Then reduce to a simmer until the carrots are very tender—about 30 minutes. Drain the carrots and place in a large bowl. Add the remaining ingredients and stir well.

Transfer the mixture to a food processor in small batches, and purée until smooth. Return the purée to a saucepan and cook over a low heat, stirring, until heated through—about 3 minutes. If you wish, serve topped with yogurt.

— Beets with Horseradish and Sour Cream —

(Serves 6–8)

The deep yin pungency of horseradish is especially beneficial for the Lungs.

6–8 medium to small beets	Boiling water
1 medium onion, finely chopped	¾ tsp salt
2 tsp prepared grated horseradish	¾ tsp freshly ground black pepper
¾ cup sour cream	

Wash the beets well, leaving the skins on together with an inch of the stem to prevent "bleeding." Cook in boiling water until tender, then let them cool and peel off the skin.

Slice the beets in ¼-inch pieces. Arrange them in a bowl and top with the chopped onion.

Blend the remaining ingredients in another bowl and spread this mixture over the beets and onion. Serve chilled.

HERBS FOR AUTUMN

During this season we need to strengthen our defenses against invading pathogens and a harsh environment. The weather becomes drier in autumn to facilitate the ripening of seeds, nuts, and grains. However, low humidity will dry out mucous membranes, making this tissue more vulnerable to viruses and bacteria. Often around the autumnal equinox there will be a wild change in weather with a quick rain- or snowstorm along with wide fluctuations in day and night temperatures, which can be followed by lovely autumn weather of warm sunny days, and cool comfortable nights. Altogether, it can be a tempestuous season of dramatic changes that take their toll on our health.

Autumn is the time to augment your immune system with Chinese herbs that reinforce the *Wei Qi*. The herbs listed below will support and protect the Lungs by supplementing qi and moisture, while reducing phlegm and warding off wind, heat, and dryness. They will reinforce the Defensive Qi, move the qi downward, and open the chest.

- *Astragalus root (Huang Qi)*—boosts *Wei Qi*, consolidates essence of Lungs and Kidneys.

- *Zhejiang fritillary bulb (Zhe Bei Mu)*—replenishes moisture and resolves phlegm.

- *Schisandra fruit (Wu Wei Zi)*—strengthens *Wei Qi* and brings it downward.

- *Platycodon root (Jie Geng)*—expels phlegm.

- *Fried anemarrhena rhizome (Chao Zhi Mu)*—moistens dryness of Lungs.

- *Chinese licorice root (Gan Cao)*—soothes throat, reduces coughing.

- *Dried ginger rhizome (Gan Jiang)*—clears wind and heat.

- *White mulberry bark (Sang Bai Pi)*—relaxes chest, moves qi downward.

- *Tangerine dried rind (Chen Pi)*—removes phlegm.

- *White mulberry leaf (Sang Ye)*—reduces heat and eases expectoration.

- *Perilla seed (Zi Suzi)*—moves phlegm out of the Lungs and sinuses.

These herbs from the Chinese *materia medica* are combined into numerous formulas that can be very helpful in fighting off colds, strengthening the Lungs and as a general qi tonic during the Metal Phase. Consult an experienced herbalist for recommendations pertaining to your particular condition. Professional advice is always recommended before using any medicinal herbs. The key to successfully treating external invasions is early action. As soon as you feel the tickle in the throat, stuffiness in the nose, or pressure in the chest or head, begin treatments with herbs, qigong, and the marvelous gargle on the next page.

A Remarkable Gargle

Here is a wonderful tip for warding off a cold. At the first sign of a sore throat, use this amazingly effective gargle solution. The sooner, the better.

Mix together the following solution:

---

1 tsp cayenne pepper   2 tbsp apple cider vinegar

1 tsp salt

To gargle, mix ¼ to ½ tsp of the solution in ½ cup of warm water. Gargle 2–3 times. Save the remaining solution in the refrigerator. Mix again and gargle every three hours until your throat feels better. It will.

CHAPTER 9

WINTER

WATER PHASE

At this season of Ultimate Yin, the foliage of plants has withered away leaving the life force ensconced in the roots; autumn's warm hazy air has been cleansed and brightened by winter's winds; flowing water slows and begins to freeze; brown meadow grass has fallen back to earth. For people, winter retracts the qi from the outer aspects of the body to be collected in the bones, Kidneys, and the LDT. Winter is both an ending and a beginning. We made decisions and took actions in autumn to rid us of negativity, harmful habits, and intemperance while retaining those positive aspects of lifestyle and mindset that form a nucleus of optimal health. Now, during winter's solitude, we have the opportunity to nurture and strengthen those qualities so they can be reborn with enhanced vigor in spring, thus carrying us further along the path of *Qigong Through the Seasons*.

The practice of Winter Qigong centers on nurturing the Kidneys, conserving and enriching *Jing*, and cultivating wisdom of the mind. The quietude of winter is an ideal time to do deep internal qigong and meditation practices for the discovery of your true nature and the seeds of spiritual awakening. This practice is rather solemn without a lot of external movement but with keen attention to the inner life. Elisabeth Rochat de la Vallée, one of the pre-eminent luminaries of Chinese scholarship, states the importance of contemplation to winter survival: "In winter you have to look after yourself, and reconsider your own life, take precautions for your own vitality, and return to your inner life for self preservation" (Larre and Rochat de la Vallée 1996, p.51).

The Chinese character for water, *shui* ("shway"), has a bold central line indicating a current of water with branching tributaries as shown in Figure 9.1. The overall impression conveys a sense of gathering energy from many directions into a single flow. Water's magnificent strength stands in contrast to its formlessness. Elusive, ungraspable, heavy, and transitory, water is a unique shape-shifter that can exist in three realms—liquid, solid, and vapor.

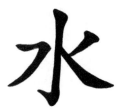

Figure 9.1: Water character

Our bodies are about 60 percent water; water covers 60 percent of the earth. The salinity of the sea is the same as our body's water. Our thirst for contacting other water-based life forms has propelled us into the universe searching for other planets that have this same primordial element of life, something we can relate to on the most fundamental level—a mirror of ourselves. From the embryonic ocean of the womb to the final dust of disintegration, water exists as the first and final elemental determinant of our life.

The Water Phase conveys stillness, clarity, and storage. In a frozen winter, the potential force of water resides in its most yin state of quietude. All the transient manifestations of life have died away and only the most essential elements remain at the core of this season and of all sentient things. Now you have the most favorable time and conditions to "return to your inner life for self preservation." Meditation practice takes you there most directly and will be the focus of Winter Qigong.

KIDNEY NETWORK

Kidneys and the urinary bladder headline the Kidney Network; other physical constituents pertain to the deepest aspects of reproduction, structure, and central control: gonads, bones, brain, and spinal cord. Functionally, the matrix of the Kidneys generates and stores *Jing*, essence, the first of the Three Treasures. It also governs reproduction and physical growth, regulates fluid dynamics, and secures the qi at the core of the body. While the Kidneys are the most Yin organs—governing water balance, sexual secretions, cerebrospinal fluid, and more—they also contain vital Kidney Yang that functions as the prime motivating force for growth and movement. The emotion of fear, when excessive or uncontrolled, has the most injurious effect on the Kidney Network. As you look around the world today, you cannot be blind to the pervasive presence of fear in humankind. The virtue of wisdom can vanquish fear. Winter Qigong gives special attention to processing the negativity of fear and cultivating the value of wisdom.

A "Water type" person will appear to have dense, large bones beneath smooth, medium-sized muscles, prominent facial bones with deep-set eyes, a long face and arms. They tend to be self-sufficient, introspective, and polite. While their scrutinizing intellect makes them knowledgeable and articulate, it can also lead to sarcasm and detachment. Water types function best with solo activities that require meticulousness, learning, and a degree of polished beauty. They make excellent scholars and researchers. Finally, and most relevant for our purposes here, they have a natural affinity for meditation. The solitary tasks of focusing on the inner landscape, maintaining mindfulness, patiently letting distractions dissolve, and then entering tranquillity, are greatly satisfying activities for these people. For this reason alone, winter may be their favorite time of year.

THE KIDNEYS IN CHINESE MEDICINE

Chinese medicine and Western medicine agree on a principle function of the Kidneys as stated in the *Su Wen*: "The Qi of the Kidneys rules Water." This includes the role of water in regulating functions of chemical composition, conversion of Vitamin D to calcitrol, and hormone production. Beyond that, Chinese medicine assigns greater roles for the essential qi of the Kidneys that revolve around the duality of Kidney Yin and Kidney Yang.

Kidney Yin energy contains our deepest source of nourishment. It generates the body's water in all of its manifestations: saliva, tears, mucus, urine, plasma, sweat, sexual secretions, and cerebrospinal and synovial fluids. The inexorable downward pull of Kidney Yin anchors the Lung Qi deep into the core of the body, refreshing every tissue with oxygen and the essence of air. We are equipped with two Kidneys and two Lungs—a unique match of paired organs—that act like poles of a battery extending from pelvis to chest. The Kidney Yin pulling downward and the Kidney Yang energy moving upward combine with the bellows action of inhalation and exhalation to efficiently transport Lung Qi throughout the body.

Kidney Yang energy has a strong vaporizing power that activates the circulation of fluids and warms the whole body. Because they are the most yin of all organs, the Kidneys have fundamental control of the water that makes life possible. Within the trunk of the body water naturally gravitates to the lowest point, which would be the region of the bladder, colon/rectum, prostate, testicles, vagina, ovaries, etc. If water stagnates in that region, we can have problems of swelling, clotting, infection, and diminished organ function. Kidney Yang warms the water and keeps it moving. This warmth enlivens the entire body and contributes to a mental and emotional sense of general comfort and contentment. Unlike the blazing fire of the Heart, Kidney Fire is a softly glowing coal buried deep in the *mingmen* area between the two organs. It keeps warm-blooded animals warm for their entire lives.

However, the Kidneys have a greater influence on our health that goes beyond water metabolism. The *Su Wen* tells us in Chapter 23 that the "The Kidneys store Essence and Will." The essence, *Jing*, is the template of our physical existence (see Chapter 1 of this book for detailed information). Because the essence holds the source of the body's yin and yang, the Kidneys have a generative relationship to the other organs in that "they hold the underlying texture of each organ's existence and are the foundation of each organ's Yin and

Yang" (Katpchuk 2000, p.84). Again, the *Su Wen* says that "the Kidneys are the root of life, the mansion of fire and water, the residence of yin and yang, the river of life and death." Put in other words, the Kidneys supply the fuel and fire that control birth, growth, maturation, aging, and death. The Will (*Zhi*, pronounced "jur"), another vital constituent of the Kidney Network, is one of the Five Spirits unique to human beings (see Chapter 7 for more about the Will). It is nourished by the Kidneys and, when cultivated with meditation and Kidney qigong practice, leads to the virtue of wisdom.

How to Practice

All qigong practice sessions should begin with "Awakening the Qi" (see page 187) and should end with "Sealing the Qi" (see page 211). This opening and closing will integrate body and mind with the energy centers and channels of qi circulation. Awakening the Qi serves as an energetic warm-up by stirring the LDT with your hands, calling to the UDT with fingertips, and warming the Kidneys with massage. Sealing the Qi concludes the practice by bringing the energy back to the LDT. In this way you do not lose the wonderful health benefits just gained.

When you finish a qigong movement, do the "Cleansing Breath": bring your feet together, stand with your arms relaxed down, your spine comfortably erect, and your eyes gazing softly into the distance. Take a deep inhalation, and then audibly and completely exhale through your mouth. Stand quietly for a few moments, intentionally point your fingers toward earth and feel the qi circulating through your body. Too often people will fidget around after doing a qigong exercise or rush into the next movement; this dissipates the energy that was just cultivated. The Cleansing Breath allows the qi to continue moving along the intended course, thus enhancing energy flow and mental equanimity. Most importantly, it brings you back to earth so that you remain rooted to this source of energy throughout the practice routine. It only takes a brief time to do, so do not neglect this important centering exercise.

Most styles of qigong have three aspects to every exercise: body movement, mental intention, and rhythmic breathing. These three factors have shifting proportions depending on the season. Winter Qigong accentuates intention. We start with the highly useful "Bear Frolic" and the intention of igniting Kidney

Yang, cultivating compassion, and practicing fearlessness. Then we switch to the yin side with "Bone Marrow Cleansing" and the intention of carrying healing energy to the center of our physical life. The final qigong exercise, "Filling the Lower *Dan Tian* to Nourish the Kidneys," is the quintessential internal method for bringing energy from earth and sky into our most important qi reservoir. However, mental intention has its most central and meaningful role in meditation, which is critically important to discovering and refining the essence of your identity and destiny. When you do the Cleansing Breath after each qigong movement, spend a little extra time standing in tranquillity, letting your awareness follow the internal circulation of your most vital energy.

WINTER QIGONG

> During winter months all things in nature wither, hide and return home. This is the time when yin dominates yang. Desires should be kept quiet and subdued. Sexual desires especially should be contained, as if keeping a happy secret. Winter season is one of conservation and storage. Without such practice the result will be injury to the kidney energy.
>
> (*The Yellow Emperor's Classic of Medicine*)

A complete discussion of sexual energy and its impact on your health is beyond the scope of this book. However, let me briefly point out the most salient aspects of sexuality as it relates to the preservation of *Jing*. Sexual function works through the actions of the Kidneys and Liver. Kidneys, testes, and ovaries store *Jing*. This fecund source of reproduction exists in limited supply within both women and men. As we saw in Chapter 1, *Jing* maintains the physical body; when it is used up, the body dies. Women lose a little *Jing* with every menstrual period; happily for them, the menopause puts an end to the depletion of this valuable Treasure. Men are not so lucky. They lose *Jing* with every ejaculation, and most men are able to ejaculate well into old age. So it becomes especially critical for men to practice sex with the aim of prolonging their physical vitality while still contributing, if they wish, to the survival of the species. The classic textbooks repeatedly admonish those who have excessive sex; that ancient wisdom remains valuable today. The Liver furnishes the blood that nourishes the vagina and uterus and enables the male erection. This blood is also important for pleasure and procreation, but because it is recycled after sex, its conservation is not as critically important to overall health.

Awakening the Qi

Warm the Dan Tian

Use your right palm to rub 36 times clockwise around your navel. Then replace your right palm with your left and rub 36 times counterclockwise.

Beat the Heavenly Drum

Cover your ears with the heels of your hands. Then tap with the fingertips on your occipital bone for about ten seconds.

Massage the Kidneys

Form loose fists with your hands, then massage up and down over your lower back 36 times.

Do Awakening the Qi only once.

Bear Frolic

The qi cultivation exercise known as the Bear Frolic comprises part of the famous and highly revered "Five Animal Frolics" developed by Hua Tuo, China's pre-eminent physician, sometime around 150 CE. The Frolics involve short sets of graceful movements based on the traits of crane, bear, monkey, deer, and tiger. This dynamic and beautiful training routine is still enjoyed by millions of practitioners throughout Asia, Europe, and North and South America. As a complete exercise system, it uses all three major aspects of qigong: movement, breathing, and intention.

Understanding the persona and innate psychic energy of each animal in the Frolics is necessary for reaping the benefits of practice. The body of the bear fills the forest with its immensity and strength. It has a deeply rooted and powerful stance with large, slightly rounded arms. The bear reigns at the top of the food chain, and thus the mind of the bear is fearless and supremely confident. And because of that attitude, the bear can also be magnanimous, benevolent, and forgiving. Humans have much to learn from the bear. When you practice the Bear Frolic, have the intention of strongly expressing the fire of Kidney Yang and equally the compassion and fearlessness that comes from the bear's inherent energy. The Bear Frolic uses all the spinal column's basic ranges of motion, thus making it a very healthy exercise for the central nervous system; and since bones and the central nervous system are principle issues for the Kidney Network, this functions as an ideal winter practice.

Bear Pushing Back

This is a wonderful toning exercise for the waist and lower back.

Stand in a slight squat with your feet wide apart. Your arms and hands assume a position with the palms up as if you were holding a large tray in each hand (students lovingly refer to this posture as "Bear Waiter") (Figure 9.2).

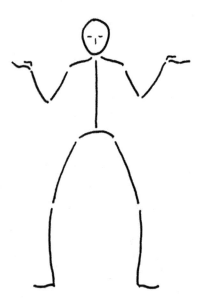

Figure 9.2: Bear Pushing Back

Inhale from the abdomen.

Exhale as you turn your torso from the waist to the left. Keep your weight 50/50 on your feet, and turn from the waist as far as is comfortable. At the same time, push your left hand back with the fingers pointing up, toward the rear. Look over your left hand and finish exhaling (Figure 9.3).

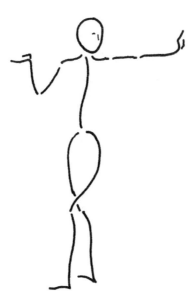

Figure 9.3: Bear Pushing Back

Inhale and turn toward the front in the starting position.

Exhale, turn your torso to the right from the waist, and push back with your right hand.

Do eight repetitions.

Bear Stretching

This movement greatly increases spinal flexibility. Think of the Bear looking for food on the ground, then expressing its strength and massive presence with open arms.

Begin by standing with your feet parallel and shoulder-width apart. Turn your right foot outward 20–30 degrees. Step forward with your left foot until the back of the heel aligns up with the tips of the right toes. Bend at the waist and bend both knees so you are in a crouch with your chest close to your left knee. Your arms are parallel and hanging down to floor, and your hands are in loose fists (Figure 9.4).

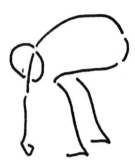

Figure 9.4: Bear Stretching

Inhale through your nose as you straighten up, as if lifting a heavy log. Keep your elbows straight and lift them up to shoulder height. As you start to bend backwards, extend your arms horizontally, keeping your hands in fists with the palms toward the sky. Look upward, open your chest, and extend your spine back (Figure 9.5).

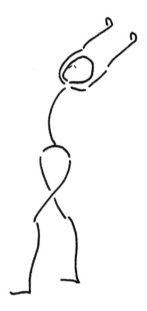

Figure 9.5: Bear Stretching

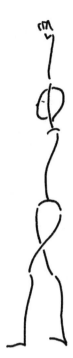

Figure 9.6: Bear Stretching

Exhale and bring your arms vertically overhead with your fingers bent like claws (Figure 9.6)

Now bend at the waist as you quickly crouch down, raking the ground with your claws, and completely exhale through your mouth. You have returned to the starting position.

Do eight repetitions.

Bear Leaning on a Wall

This movement mimics the bear's rolling and swaying gait; it has a pleasant rhythm with a calm demeanor. Mentally lead the qi from your feet, up through your trunk, and out through your hands. Find a nice symmetrical cadence in moving from side to side. Stand with your feet shoulder-width apart, and toes pointing forward. Your hands are at the LDT with the palms up (Figure 9.7).

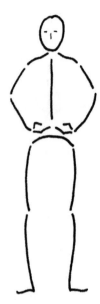

Figure 9.7: Bear Leaning on a Wall

Inhale as you shift your weight onto your right leg, raise your hands up to your chest, drop your elbows, so your forearms are vertical and parallel, and turn your palms so they are facing outward in front of your shoulders (Figure 9.8).

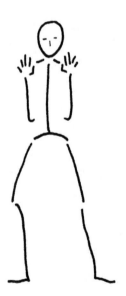

Figure 9.8: Bear Leaning on a Wall

Still inhaling, pivot on the heel of your left foot so the toes turn to the left, your body turns to the left, and your palms also face left (Figure 9.9). Your weight remains on your right leg, with the right foot still facing forward. Your right knee is slightly bent, your left knee is straight.

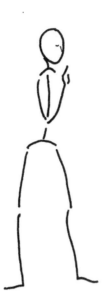

Figure 9.9: Bear Leaning on a Wall

Exhale as your weight shifts from your right leg onto your left leg, and your body leans to the left, as your hands press over your left leg, as if you were leaning on a wall (Figure 9.10). Your right knee is straight, your left knee is bent.

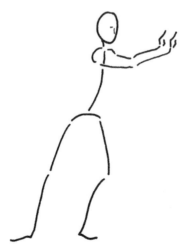

Figure 9.10: Bear Leaning on a Wall

Inhale as you shift back onto your right leg, and your hands come down to the LTD (Figure 9.11).

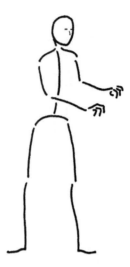

Figure 9.11: Bear Leaning on a Wall

Continue inhaling and pivot on the heel of your left foot so the toes point to the front. Still inhaling, shift your weight onto your left foot as your right foot pivots on the heel and turns to the right. Your weight is on your right leg as your hands lift up from the LDT to your chest with the palms facing forward (Figure 9.12).

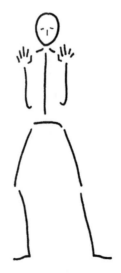

Figure 9.12: Bear Leaning on a Wall

Shift your weight onto your left leg, and turn your body to the right, with your hands still in front of your shoulders. Your left knee is bent, your right knee is straight (Figure 9.13).

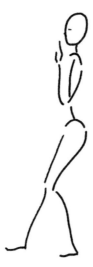

Figure 9.13: Bear Leaning on a Wall

Exhale as your weight shifts onto your right leg. Your body leans to the right, and your hands press over your right leg as if you were leaning on a wall.

Do eight repetitions (four each side).

Bear Stretching

Repeat Bear Stretching exactly like you did the first time (see pages 190–91), only step forward with your right foot instead of your left. Turn your left foot outward 20–30 degrees. Do the same movements, with the same intention.

Do eight repetitions.

Bear Growling

Now we really rev up the Yang Qi of the bear. The attitude is fierce—passionate, but with underlying benevolence. You must audibly growl for this exercise, which is quite difficult for some people. But remember, it's a "frolic" so have fun! The movement efficiently tones and strengthens the lateral abdominal muscles, which are too often neglected in most exercise programs. Keep these points in mind: feel the effect of growling on your body; every bear has its own voice. Feel the rootedness in your legs and the strength in your torso. Then let the growl of fearlessness transform into a manifestation of the bear's benevolence by not dropping the rock. Again, this exercise requires an attitude.

Stand with your feet more than shoulder-width apart. Your hands are at the level of the LDT with the palms up as if holding a large rock. Your arms are slightly rounded. Bend down from the waist.

Inhale as you twist your body to the left so your hands are a few inches above your left foot (Figure 9.14).

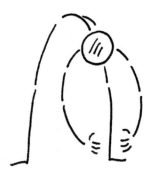

Figure 9.14: Bear Growling

Continue inhaling as you straighten up, rotating your torso so your right elbow points skyward (feel the stretch along your right ribcage), while your left arm supports the "rock" (Figure 9.15).

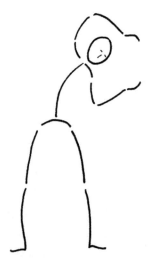

Figure 9.15: Bear Growling

Keep inhaling and lifting, as if going around a clock face, until your hands are overhead at 12 o'clock (Figure 9.16).

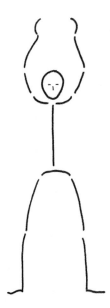

Figure 9.16: Bear Growling

Exhale with a growl and rotate your body to the right, bringing the rock aggressively downward around the clockface toward your right foot as if you were just about to drop it—the growl is to let all the animals in the forest know that you are at the top of the food chain and could crush them with your rock. However, you do not, because you are magnanimous and possess the benevolence of a fearless monarch. Feel how your body and mind are replete with the incredible power of the bear. Finish exhaling as you carry the rock to the right and down to the six o'clock position. Continue down and to the left as you *inhale*.

Do this four times one way, then reverse directions and do it four times the other way.

Bear Offering

Finally, we come into the abode of the bear's Yin Qi, where compassion and goodwill are nurtured. This transition from yang aggressiveness to yin kindness is smooth and delicate. Many people find this exercise elicits an emotional response in them because it can be done with loving intention to many different people. And love has many layers of complexity. The movement is very short; however, the intention reaches far into space.

You can send Bear Offering to three different types: first, send the offering to two individuals that you know and love—in your immediate family or close circle of friends. Second, send the offering to two groups of people that you know about but have no emotional connection with—perhaps you have heard of their plight in the news media. Third, send the offering to individuals or groups whom you find it very difficult to agree with—this works especially well for politicians, extremists, and harsh manipulators. The purpose of the exercise hinges on finding the preciously common thread of humanity that runs far beneath appearances and actions.

Stand with your feet shoulder-width apart. Your hands are at the LDT, with the palms up and the middle fingertips touching. Think of two individuals or two groups of people to whom you would like to make an offering. The offering should come from the magnanimous power of the bear: compassion, goodwill, gratitude, charity, or whatever offering you want to make that contributes to love and peace throughout the world.

Inhale and think of taking the offering into your body.

Exhale slowly and turn your body to the left, extending your left arm out to the side (Figure 9.17). Your right little finger touches the inside of your left elbow, and both palms are up as if offering a gift. Your feet do not move. Mentally, project this offering to the receiver of your choice. This is the first repetition.

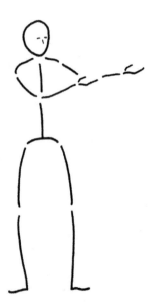

Figure 9.17: Bear Offering

Inhale slowly and return to the starting position. Again, bring the offering into your body.

Exhale slowly, turn your body to the right, and send this offering out with your mind-Heart-breath to the recipients. That is the second repetition.

Do eight repetitions (four each side).

Bone Marrow Cleansing

Bone Marrow Cleansing, *Xi Sui Jing*, is an ancient practice that has been attributed to Bodhidharma, the fifth-century Buddhist sage who resided for a time at Shaolin Temple. However, academic research both in China and the West does not support this claim that Bodhidharma taught this practice to the monks. There are many variations of Bone Marrow Cleansing and the original source may be lost in the dim light of antiquity. I maintain that this practice exists today because practitioners experience a state of profound well being created by the synergy of celestial, terrestrial and human energy fields accessed in the exercise.

These exercises focus primarily on accumulating the qi from nature and circulating it through the marrow to wash the innermost qi repositories with fresh energy from heaven and earth. In Chinese medicine the term "marrow" refers to the bones, brain, and, by extension, the spinal cord. You have seen that these structures relate closely to the Kidney Network. Any disorder of these *Jing*-related elements can be treated with qigong, acupuncture, and those herbs that have an effect on the Kidneys (see Kaptchuk 2000, pp.351–2). This highly revered practice covers multiple existential dimensions: mountain strength, spiritual structure, celestial power, wise illumination, and finally the skeleton of your body. Because the practice touches on so many facets of being human, Bone Marrow Cleansing universally benefits everyone. Many of my students claim this as one of their all-time favorite practices.

Bone Marrow Cleansing as a *neigong* exercise directs qi inward to its deepest recesses and pathways. It requires subtle but dedicated attention to reach this most essential undercurrent of life. *Neigong* should be done with a sense of quietness, peace, and awareness—as if you were seeing and feeling the inner movement of an energy that is almost palpable. Think of qi as a force with the potential to become a substance.

Bone marrow and the Kidneys are storage areas for the *Jing*. The first directive in the process of inner alchemy is to "transform the *Jing* into *Qi*." You can use the energies of yin/earth and yang/heaven to facilitate this transformation, thus beginning the human odyssey toward well-being and ultimately spiritual awakening.

Wisdom Posture

Stand with your feet together and your hands at your sides. Step to the side with your left foot.

Inhale as you lift your hands up to the LDT, as if encircling a ball, with the palms facing your body (Figure 9.18).

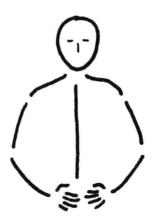

Figure 9.18: Wisdom Posture

Exhale and lightly put your attention on the LDT.

Inhale as you lift your hands up to chest level, place your palms together, and bring your hands to your chest with the thumbs touching your body (Figure 9.19).

Exhale and relax with your knees slightly bent.

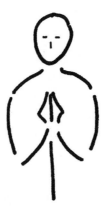

Figure 9.19: Wisdom Posture

Let everything relax to your very bones. Maintain this posture as your mind becomes calm and your body feels as strong as a mountain. Feel that the universe is within you. Feel the energy of heaven and earth collecting inside your body as if it were creating a great centripetal force. Let the eternal wisdom of nature fill your body and mind. Be quietly still like this, breathing calmly, for a few minutes. Think of yourself being a monumental summit with your head in the clouds; your arms are the forested slopes, your feet are straddling a vast distance on earth.

Now lower your hands to your sides and step back to center with your left foot.

Do this exercise once.

Building the Foundation

Step to the left with arms at sides.

Inhale as you lift your arms out laterally and up to shoulder height (Figure 9.20). Your palms are facing the earth. Be relaxed and open.

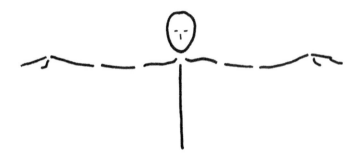

Figure 9.20: Building the Foundation

Exhale and bend your knees as you bring your hands down to about hip level (Figure 9.21). (Bring your hands down with a sense that you are pushing two large balls under water, feeling a slight resistance to the sinking hands. Imagine that you are laying down material to build a foundation for a temple or church—something that has spiritual connotations.)

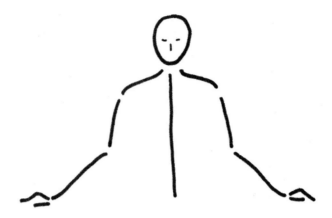

Figure 9.21: Building the Foundation

Inhale as you stand up and let your arms float back up to shoulder height as if they were wings. The movement is light and effortless.

Exhale as you bend your knees and push down. Imagine you are laying down another layer of building material for the temple. You just did two repetitions.

Do eight repetitions in total, then step back to the center with your left foot.

Plucking Stars

Begin with feet together, hands relaxed at sides. Move the left foot laterally so the feet are now about shoulder width apart. In this exercise, do not try to coordinate your breathing with the movements. Let the breath come and go naturally. Always remain relaxed and focused inward.

Place the back of your left hand over the center of your lower back, which is the area of the Kidneys and *mingmen* (acupuncture point GV4 in the middle of the lumbar spine). Raise your right hand out from your side and slowly up over your head until the palm is a few inches above *baihui* (GV20) at the crown of your head (Figure 9.22). Think of *baihui*.

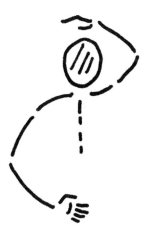

Figure 9.22: Plucking Stars

Now turn your right palm upward and reach toward heaven (Figure 9.23)

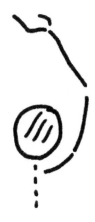

Figure 9.23: Plucking Stars

Now "pluck" the energy of a star as you turn your hand over and slowly bring it down the front of your body with the palm toward the earth (Figure 9.24). Think of bringing the qi of that star into your *brain* and then down through your *spinal column*.

When your right hand comes to your belly, place the thumb on your navel and the palm against your abdomen. The left hand remains against the lower back.

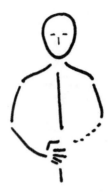

Figure 9.24: Plucking Stars

Think of holding the qi in the LDT between your two hands. Stand quietly for three breaths. Relax. Look inward. Don't be concerned about placing your rear hand exactly over GV4. The hand is broad enough to cover this area and that's all that is needed—it brings the celestial energy to the *area*, not to a specific acupuncture point.

Now place your right hand over *mingmen* and raise the left hand out from your side and slowly up over your head until the palm is a few inches above *baihui* (GV20) at the crown of your head. Turn the hand over and pluck a star. Bring that celestial energy down through the spinal column and to the belly. Do a total of four repetitions. Finish by stepping back to the center with feet together.

The Sage

Do not try to coordinate your breathing with the movements in this exercise.

Step to the left and turn your palms so they are facing forward (Figure 9.25).

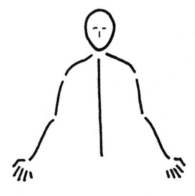

Figure 9.25: The Sage

Slowly lift your arms laterally to shoulder height. When you begin the movement, first think of your little fingers coming up, then your ring fingers, next your middle fingers, then your index fingers, and finally your thumbs. Feel that your hands are filled with qi.

Stand with your arms wide and your palms facing forward. Your fingers should be extended so that the *laogong* points in the center of your palms are open (Figure 9.26). Relax.

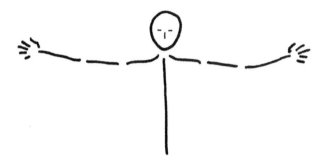

Figure 9.26: The Sage

Think big. Feel yourself filling all of the space around you. Have the magnitude of the Wisdom Posture (see page 200), but instead of a solid mountain, think of yourself as a luminous being with a barely perceptible form. You are so light and porous that all forms of energy—light, wind, and cosmic radiation—pass through you and are amplified as they whirl out into space with colorful contrails of numinous energy. You are now a centrifugal force. Let the alchemical transformation of yin from the earth and yang from the heavens radiate the qi of your being outward. The sum of this energy supports your body in space, your arms are effortlessly expansive, your head is held high, your whole body is vibrant with color. And you are completely relaxed.

Stand this way for two to three minutes. Let the qi flow. Then lower your hands to your sides and step back to center.

Washing the Bone Marrow

Step to the left. Lift your hands to just below your navel with the palms up and fingers pointing toward each other (Figure 9.27). Pause and take one slow, gentle breath.

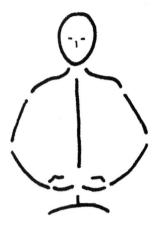

Figure 9.27: Washing the Bone Marrow

Now lift your hands up to your chest, and turn them over so the palms are facing heaven as you push up and forward away from your head (Figure 9.28). Take one slow breath.

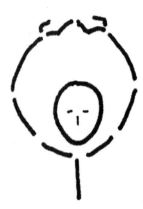

Figure 9.28: Washing the Bone Marrow

Now turn your hands so the palms are facing earth, and bring them over the crown of your head (Figure 9.29). Think of the *laogong* points connecting with *baihui*. Take a long, slow breath and feel the energy between hands and the top of your head.

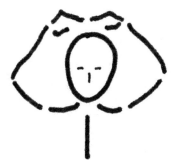

Figure 9.29: Washing the Bone Marrow

Very slowly bring your hands down in front of your body. Let your breath come and go naturally. Don't try to time your breath with the movement. Just breathe gently. Go slowly. This will take several breath cycles.

As your hands slowly descend, think of your skeleton. First, think of the long bones in your hands and arms. Look at them as if you were seeing an X-ray, and imagine looking into the bone marrow cavities. Then think of the ribs. See them as your hands pass by. With your mind, bring fresh, clear qi into the marrow cavities of all the bones your hands are passing by. Feel that all impurities are being drained away by this healing energy.

When your hands are at hip level, straighten your elbows and point your fingers toward the earth (Figure 9.30).

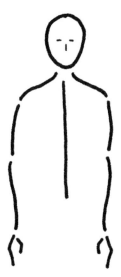

Figure 9.30: Washing the Bone Marrow

Mentally lead the qi down through the center of the long bones in your legs. Take your time. The femurs are huge repositories of bone marrow. Relax. Look inward. Finish by taking qi out through the little bones of your toes.

Step back to center. Remain still, letting your hands hang naturally at your sides, with the fingers slightly extended down. Imagine fresh, pure qi streaming through the marrow cavities in your skull, hands, ribs, vertebrae, arms, pelvis, legs, and feet.

Stand quietly and breathe softly for a minute.

Filling the Lower *Dan Tian* to Nourish the Kidneys

The LDT functions as an alchemical stove. It has a diffuse boundary going from the lower abdomen, down to the perineum, up the lower back, and forward beneath the diaphragm. The essence of food and air becomes transformed inside the LDT into the qi that circulates through the meridian system. The Kidneys are located close to the LDT and have the primary role of being "the foundation of each organ's yin and yang" (Kaptchuk 2000, p.84). That's a big responsibility. Without the Water and Fire of the Kidneys, all of the other organs would wither away.

This exercise brings the healing qi from earth and sky into the "*Taiji Axis*" (see Chapter 1 for detailed information), then down to the Heart where it mixes with the qi of the chest, and then down to the LDT for purification and storage. Filling the Lower *Dan Tian* to Nourish the Kidneys has a rich potential for bringing into the body the vital healing energies of terrestrial, celestial, and human sources.

This is the premier qigong exercise for Winter Qigong. Movement is kept to a minimum, and mental intention is elevated to prime importance; it brings the limitless energy of the outside world into the most interior nucleus of personal existence. And then it powerfully packs the treasured qi into the bedrock reservoir of vitality, there to be slowly refined and nourished for self-preservation through the long season of Ultimate Yin.

Stand with your feet about shoulder-width apart, and your hands down with the palms near the lateral sides of your thighs.

Inhale slowly as you lift your arms laterally in a big arc, with your palms up, to an overhead position with palms touching (Figure 9.31). Think of bringing in fresh qi from the earth and from the sky. Then compress this qi between your hands. Imagine that you are consolidating and transforming raw elements into a priceless jewel.

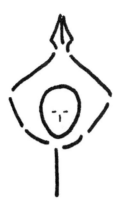

Figure 9.31: Filling the LDT to Nourish the Kidneys

Exhale very slowly through your nose as your hands, in prayer position, come down your body's midline to your chest (Figure 9.32).

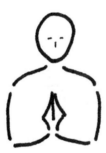

Figure 9.32: Filling the LDT to Nourish the Kidneys

Think of bringing the qi gem down the *Taiji Axis* and into your Heart. Although your hands move in front of your body, the energy is brought down the internal channel. Still exhaling, turn your hands over into a diamond shape with the fingers pointing down, thumbs up, and palms against your body (Figure 9.33).

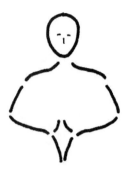

Figure 9.33: Filling the LDT to Nourish the Kidneys

Continue to exhale as the qi comes down the *Taiji Axis* and flows into the LDT. Finish the exhalation with your thumbs at your navel and your palms against the LDT. Relax.

Inhale and turn your hands so that the palms are facing each other, with the fingers still pointing down, then move your hands apart—just out to hip-width. This is a short inhalation.

Exhale and bring your palms toward each other until they are almost touching. Think of packing the valuable energy into the LDT for storage (Figure 9.34).

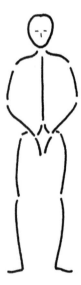

Figure 9.34: Filling the LDT to Nourish the Kidneys

At the end of this short exhalation, drop your hands to your sides and relax your shoulders.

Do eight repetitions.

Sealing the Qi

Whole Body Tapping

Use your palms to tap over each arm, your trunk, outer legs, inner legs, abdomen, and lower back (use your fists on your back). Do this three times.

Arms Horizontal

Put your arms straight out to the sides, with your fingers pointing up, for one breath.

Heaven and Earth

Inhale and lift your hands laterally and then overhead, with the palms pointing to heaven. Rise up on your toes and hold your breath for a few seconds. Slowly exhale, lower your heels, and with palms facing the earth, lower your hands to the LDT.

Seal

Cover the LDT with the palm of your right hand. Place the palm of your left hand over your right hand with the thumb tucked under your right hand. Stand quietly for three breaths.

Do Sealing the Qi only once.

WINTER MEDITATION

Seven Stars on the Microcosmic Orbit Meditation

The primary circuit of qi circulation consists of the Conception Vessel and the Governing Vessel. These two meridians form an orbit of energy flowing down the front of the body, up the spine and over the head. The anterior Conception Vessel (CV) moves the Yin Qi. The posterior Governing Vessel (GV) carries Yang Qi. These two meridians, when united as one, form the Microcosmic Orbit for transporting the qi after it has emerged from the LDT. When this Microcosmic Orbit becomes replete with abundant and unobstructed qi, it releases this energy into the 12 regular meridians, which then carry it to every tissue and cell in the body. Along the Microcosmic Orbit there are seven acupuncture points that stand out as critical vortexes, which have vital influences on adjacent regions of the body as shown in Figure 9.35. You can augment the functional energy of a point by putting your mind and breath on it for a short time, giving it your full attention, and then moving on to the next point. In this way you nourish the power in each point while also enhancing the overall circulation through the Microcosmic Orbit.

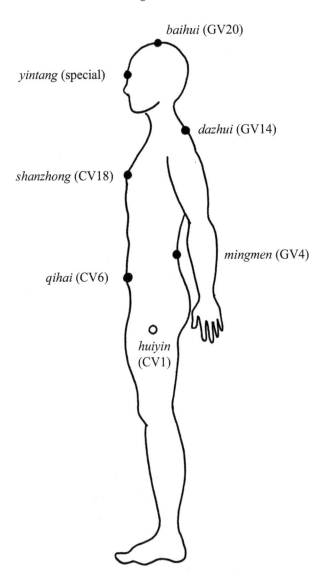

Figure 9.35: Seven Stars on the Microcosmic Orbit Meditation

Use Figure 9.35 as a reference for point locations. You do not have to be precisely on the point; rather, you use meditative placement of your intention to cover the region *around* the acupuncture point. The names and numbers are included because Seven Stars Meditation is traditionally indicated in this way, and it is good to get as close to the point as possible.

Begin in a comfortably seated position. The instructions tell you to take three breaths at each star. You may take more or fewer, but if you are new to this meditation, it is better to maintain about the same duration at each point along the way so that a rhythmical flow goes through the Microcosmic Orbit. Eventually you may want to do it, like I do, without counting any breaths, just letting your intuition tell you when to stay and when to move on. If your perception of internal energy balance is well developed, you will know which points/regions need more attention than others and will adjust your time there accordingly.

Put your attention on *huiyin*, CV1, at the center of the perineum. *Inhale* and gently contract and lift this point upward. Then *exhale* and relax. Take three breaths.

Now put your attention on *mingmen*, GV4, at the center of the lower back. *Inhale* (no muscle contraction) and think of taking qi into your body at this point. *Exhale* and let the energy sink into the Kidneys and *mingmen*. Take three breaths, staying focused on the point.

Move your attention up to *dazhui*, GV14, at the base of your neck. *Inhale* into this area. *Exhale* and relax. Let your shoulders and neck relax. Breathe slowly and gently three times.

With your mind, move the qi to the top of the head at *baihui*, GV20. This point is for connecting with the qi of heaven and enlivening your Spirit. *Inhale* and *exhale* slowly. Imagine your head is suspended from above by a golden thread. Take three breaths.

Now, bring your attention to *yintang* (special point) between the eyebrows. Relax here. *Inhale* and open this portal to the UDT. *Exhale* and let the qi sink inward. Take three breaths.

Then move down to *shanchong*, CV18, located the width of eight fingers below the clavicles. To find it, align four fingers of each hand horizontally from the clavicles to the sternum—CV18 is just below the lowest finger. *Inhale* to the MDT. *Exhale*. Let your Heart open. Remain here for three breaths.

Finally, rest your mind at *qihai*, CV6, the "ocean of energy." *Inhale* and *exhale* like slow waves ebbing and flowing through the LDT. Let go of all thoughts. Just breathe here for a few minutes.

Lake and Geyser

Three major energy centers in the body are called the *dan tians*, "elixir field," or "the place where internal medicine is cultivated." In terms of Western anatomy they are located in the gut, heart, and brain. The *dan tians* are reservoirs of powerful healing forces and the abode of the Three Treasures (see Chapter 1 for details).

The LDT, as the primary reservoir of qi, corresponds to *Jing*—the earth and sexuality. This *dan tian* functionally helps heal the body by way of refining the *Jing* and cultivating qi. The MDT houses the HeartMind (see Chapter 7), which develops over time from merging the feeling-self and the thinking-self; with further practice, the *Qi* is refined into *Shen* and then healthy emotions and human compassion flourish. The UDT is the palace of the *Shen*. The *Shen*, or Spirit, develops from the joining of the HeartMind with higher consciousness and universal wisdom. The cultivation of this uniquely human Treasure epitomizes spiritual awakening.

The *Taiji Axis* connects the three *dan tians* into a single pathway of ascending and Descending Qi. This thoroughfare of qi transport lies at the body's most cavernous recess, and because of that interiority it correlates with the deeply inward movement of Winter's Qi, making this season a perfect time to contact and engage with the *Taiji Axis*. The practicality of fulfilling the prime directive of qigong—to transform *Jing* into qi, refine qi into *Shen*, awaken *Shen* and return to the Void—takes place along the central *taiji* channel by way of the Lake and Geyser Meditation. What really makes this method special is that the energetic flow transforms from ascending, to simultaneously up and down, and finally to descending, which matches the idea that spiritual awakening eventually leads one back to living in the world with peace and contentment.

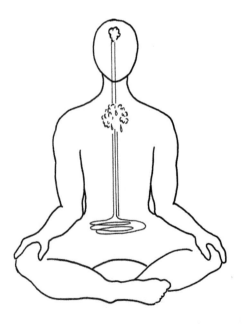

Figure 9.36: Lake and Geyser Meditation

Begin in a comfortably seated position.

Put your attention on the LDT. Relax and look inward. The LDT is like a placid lake with crystal-clear water embraced by a circular shore. Breathe slowly and gaze upon the lake. Notice how your breath creates small ripples on the water. When you inhale, see the ripples come toward the center in concentric circles, getting smaller toward the middle. When you exhale, the ripples move outward and disappear on the calm surface of the water. Inhale, and the little waves move toward the center. Exhale, and they relax.

The moving force behind the waves is qi. Your mind and your breath control the movement of qi. See how the waves at the center of the circle rise upward when you breathe in, like a spout rising above the surface. Your mind is lifting the water (Figure 9.36). When you breathe out, your mind brings the water back to stillness in the LDT. With each inhalation the water rises up further, getting taller like a fountain.

Breathe like this for a little while, gently directing the rise and fall of the qi.

Now, move your attention to the *MDT* in your chest. See how each breath brings the water fountain higher up, toward the MDT; and when you exhale the water returns to the LDT. Rising up, flowing down. The water becomes warmer as it moves between the two *dan tians*. It rises with more vigor, getting stronger.

Now see this rising column of water become a geyser, surging upward and billowing out into the MDT, covering this space with a fine spray of pure, clear water. Then the geyser drops down to its source in the LDT.

Inhale, lifting the water up. Exhale, letting it down. See how this beautiful geyser rises up into your chest and bursts forth with shimmering droplets of water. Then they gently return to the LDT. The geyser gets larger until its dome fills the entire MDT, bathing this place with warm, iridescent energy.

Relax and gently breathe here for a couple of minutes. Use your mind to lead the qi *between the LDT and the MDT*.

The geyser of qi becomes heated with the movement of your mind. This warmth releases steam that rises to the *UDT* in your head. Feel this softly billowing steam fill the UDT as you breathe in. Then your long, slow exhalation drains the steam all the way down to the LDT. As you inhale, the water swells up to your chest, and steam rises into the UDT. It is like a white healing mist, filling the space with pure energy and then gently returning to its source in the placid lake.

As you breathe in, the water rises from the lake, steaming like a geyser, and the vapors rise to the UDT.

Relax your mind. Relax your body. Just breathe: breathe in; breathe out. Feel this warm healing mist cleansing the UDT. As you relax further into your breathing, feel the rising and falling of the qi.

Now, look closely…see that this fountain of water is now a continuous column where the water simultaneously goes up and down without end. It's a scintillating column of water glittering with energy, bringing the three *dan tians* into harmony, into the present moment where the entire *dan tian* axis is filled with qi. Relax and imagine that you are bathing within this column of gleaming energy.

Soon this glistening column of water begins to lose its form. And now it's a mass of sparkles, like a starry sky extending from your belly, through your torso, and into your head—a sparkling array of energy.

Just breathe and relax. Feel the spaciousness of the *dan tians* for a little while.

And now, as you gaze into this starry scene, as you watch these twinkling droplets of water, they begin to drop downward, gently floating back down to the LDT. All of the energy returns to the placid lake. Your breath becomes quiet and still.

All of the energy flows back down into the lake, returning to the source.

This descending energy comes in little waves, flowing into the lake, moving toward the center.

All of your energy is gathering in this bottomless lake.

Let your mind relax. Let your breath become quiet—almost imperceptible like the embryonic breath.

You are floating upon the lake. It's a sea of qi, a boundless ocean of energy.

This is the source of good health, happiness, and tranquility. Live here.

Three Stars of the Lower *Dan Tian*

This short meditation utilizes three of the seven points on the Microcosmic Orbit to specifically energize the LDT, our principal concern in winter. The *qihai* ("Sea of Qi") and *mingmen* ("Gate of Life") are extremely important points used in acupuncture treatments as well as in qigong practice. Their yin–yang polarity creates a horizontally oriented direction of qi flow, which is quite unique in the meridian system. This level line demarcates the upper and lower parts of the physical body. *Huiyin* ("Gathering Yin") functions as the most essential yin point on the trunk of the body because it is at the bottom of the torso and is the lower pole of the all-important *Taiji Axis*. Please see Figure 9.35 (page 212) for the location of the three stars that surround the LDT.

During the wintertime, the qi retracts from the outer aspects of the body to collect in the bones and in the LDT. While qi circulates continuously throughout the meridian system, there is also an accumulation of qi in this lower region, much like a deep, quiet pool of water within a flowing river. This natural process of gathering energy should be encouraged if we want to maintain good health. The LDT collects qi like a reservoir.

When the qi has filled the LTD, it then flows out into the Microcosmic Orbit and on to the major meridians of the body. Thus all qi circulation is dependent on the LDT first becoming replete with qi.

Begin in a comfortably seated position.

Allow the breath to come slowly and to sink into the LDT. Think of *qihai*. Look inward, and see a vast body of water going all the way to the horizon. Waves ebb and flow on the water. You want this "Sea of Qi" to become still and tranquil. Your breath becomes slower. The waves start to settle down.

Now, move your attention to *huiyin*. This is the gathering place of the Yin Qi that connects with the energy of earth and relates to the first Treasure, the *Jing*. It pertains to rootedness and sexuality. Breathe gently into *huiyin*. Let the stillness at the surface of the water drop peacefully down to *huiyin*. This is the bottom of the LDT. Feel the substance of this area. As you gently breathe, let all of the qi energy from the body sink to this point.

Now, with your mind, move the qi from *huiyin* through the sacrum up to *mingmen*. Breathe into *mingmen* and fill this area with qi. *Mingmen* is the Gate of Life, the source of Yang Qi. As you breathe into *mingmen*, feel the area becoming warmer, like an ember of fire. Use your mind to warm the breath and let it flow into *mingmen*. Feel this movement bring the Yang Qi into the LDT, like a warm bubbling pool of water.

Now, bring the qi from *mingmen* forward through your body toward *qihai*. See this as a slow tide of warm qi flowing through the LDT from the back to the front. Breathe gently and deeply as the tide of energy comes into *qihai*. Continue to consciously circulate the qi through the three stars on the LDT for as long as you wish.

Making Fear Disappear

Fear has a wide range of emotional manifestations, from just a vague uneasiness, or a depressed attitude, to a reoccurring avoidance of something threatening. Fear can grow as a feeling of impending doom. Ultimately, it can result in a full-blown paralysis of mind and body. Chinese medicine tells us that fear will exhaust the Yang Qi of the kidneys, which is the energy that fuels our basic "fight or flight" reaction to fearful situations. If this reaction is prolonged, or reoccurs frequently, it leads to burnout of the adrenal glands and a definite decline in our health.

Fear is everywhere. Daily newspapers and media reports thrive on it. Politicians use it as a tool to force their agenda on the public. Personal relationships may be defined by it. Self-esteem may be hampered by it. Fear comes in a variety of sizes and colors.

Our reaction to any situation—past, present, or future—begins in our mind. Many fears result from our predictions of what will happen in the future. Often times we think the worst case scenario will come from what we are afraid of at the moment. Most fears are exaggerations that don't come true. The great American humorist Mark Twain said that some of the worse things in his life never even happened.

People have a unique ability to talk to themselves. We spend much of our time carrying on an internal dialogue about the past or the future. And, because we are mostly unaware of our true nature, this inner talk usually comes out more negative than positive. It makes fear more real than it is. Meditation can help us stop this internal babble and come to rest in a place of stillness where we can understand the true nature of things. And then we may know that what we often fear is, in the end, not really to be feared at all.

Begin by sitting quietly in mindfulness, just breathing and becoming aware of your breath.

Now, give a name to what you fear the most at this time. Name this fear with only a word or two that really gets to the heart of it. Put it in big bold letters on the screen of your mind. Relax, and just look at the word.

Imagine that you are observing a snowy field in nature. Maybe it is late in the afternoon with that beautifully subtle, long-reaching light of winter. And there on the edge of the field you see a bank of drifted snow in the pale sunlight.

On this white bank of snow you see—written in clear black letters—the words of what you fear.

Look closely. Breathe slowly. Take a minute to just observe the letters of your fear.

Now, use your mind to direct your breath out to this drift of fear. Breathe deeply with long exhalations. Let your exhalations blow across the words in the snow. As you sit and calmly breathe in and out, don't have any thoughts about the fear, just see the words. Breathe slowly, deeply.

Feel your warm breath go out to the words on the snow bank.

Soon you see how the fear begins to melt away as you continue to mindfully project the power of your breath onto the fear.

Eventually there is nothing left to fear.

Figure 9.37: Making Fear Disappear Meditation

SUGGESTIONS FOR WINTER PRACTICE

You can use the following components of the Winter Qigong Practice to build your personal two-part program of qigong and meditation. Be serious, but enjoy the time you are taking to do something good for yourself.

1. *Qigong*: Awakening the Qi; Bear Frolic; Bone Marrow Cleansing; Filling the Lower *Dan Tian* to Nourish the Kidneys; Sealing the Qi.

2. *Meditation*: Three Stars of the Lower *Dan Tian*; Seven Stars on the Microcosmic Orbit; Lake and Geyser; Making Fear Disappear.

For a complete practice, do Awakening the Qi, Bear Frolic, Bone Marrow Cleansing, Filling the Lower *Dan Tian*, and Sealing the Qi. This takes about 10–12 minutes. Add to this one of the meditations. If you are doing a morning practice, it is good to begin with meditation. If it is an evening practice, it is good to end with meditation.

You may do the qigong practice one day and one of the meditations on the next day. Most practitioners only do one of the meditations in a single practice period.

You may also do qigong in the morning and a meditation in the evening. This would be in keeping with the predominant energy at that time of day/evening.

Make a commitment to do at least some part of the practice every day. Having a regular practice is more important than the length of a session. Practicing at the same time each day is helpful. The hardest part is simply getting started that day. Once you awaken the qi, you will be glad that you are there.

FOODS AND HERBS FOR WINTER

You can to some extent control your internal thermostat by what you eat. Foods have a general influence on the body's temperature: they are either warming or cooling. The following food groups are warming: grains, seeds, nuts, legumes, cheese, eggs, seafood, poultry, and meat—especially wild game. In a similar way, the method of preparation also affects the heating power of food. Baked, fried, roasted, or broiled food will impart more heat to your body than steamed, sautéed, dried, or raw food.

The *salty* flavor correlates to the Kidney Network. Generally this ubiquitous flavor overwhelms the typical diet. But salt is as essential to our health as seawater is to the ocean, so the most natural sources of this flavor will be miso, soy sauce, and seaweeds. Of the grains, millet and barley seem to have a higher salt content than other cereals. You probably already have enough salt in your diet, so don't add more just because it is winter.

Some of the best plant foods for the Kidney include the following: black beans, black sesame seeds, corn, parsley, millet, nuts, quinoa, and wild rice. The Kidneys, because they harbor the *Jing* and are directors of physical growth, respond very well to high-quality pork and wild game. Venison is one of the most yang foods you can eat; the protein is easily digestible and very low in fat.

Nuts top the list of favorable winter foods. Chinese dietary medicine views nuts as beneficial because, in addition to having excellent nutrients, they are seeds. And seeds contain *Jing*, the generative essence of the plant. *Jing* drives the growth of any species, whether plant or animal. When we eat nuts and other seeds the *Jing* contained in those foods has a positive influence on the *Jing* within us through the resonance of the generative energetic systems of both species. We not only absorb essential nutrients from the plants we eat, we also obtain *Jing* and the bioenergetic nutrients that feed our essential base of structural growth and maintenance.

GO NUTS

Nuts and seeds are finally getting the accolade from Western science that has so long been granted to them by Chinese medicine. Now everyone acknowledges them as nutritional powerhouses containing a potent mix of protein, essential fatty acids, vitamin E, minerals, and monounsaturated fats. Some people refer to them as "the perfect food."

Over 30 studies have shown serum cholesterol and triglyceride levels were favorably reduced when nuts were included in the diet. This got the attention of the US Food and Drug Administration (FDA). In 2003, the FDA made this statement: "Scientific evidence suggests but does not prove that eating 1.5 ounces (42g) per day of most nuts as part of a diet low in saturated fat and cholesterol, may reduce the risk of heart disease. See nutrition information for fat content."[2]

Nuts and seeds have such a positive effect on blood pressure that they have become part of the highly regarded DASH Diet for controlling hypertension. This effect may result from the fact that nuts offer excellent sources of calcium, magnesium, and potassium. Some findings suggest that, because they absorb slowly, eating nuts may lower the Glycemic Index (GI) of a meal—the rate that food is converted to glucose. A low GI provides a stable supply of glucose without the wild swings that come from refined foods. That bodes well for people with hypoglycemia, diabetes, or obesity.

The wealth of nutrients in nuts makes them calorie dense. This worries some people concerned about their weight. However, including a handful of nuts in the daily diet may actually expedite weight loss. In addition to all the good things, nuts give people a sense of satiety. Perhaps snacking on a few nuts instead of eating celery sticks will help people stay on a weight loss program and avoid serial dieting.

Researchers at Brigham and Women's Hospital and the Harvard School of Public Health found that three times as many people trying to lose weight were able to stick to a Mediterranean-style, moderate-fat weight loss diet that included nuts, peanuts, and peanut butter, vs. the traditionally recommended low-fat diet (McManus, Antinoro, and Sacks 2001).

I suggest a daily serving of 1½ oz of nuts (2–3 tbsp). Take a look at the following range of healthy ingredients in a variety of nuts:

- *Almonds*: A 1oz (28g) serving is about 24 nuts with 6g protein, 160 calories, and 9g monosaturated fat. Almonds are loaded with Vitamin E (an antioxidant that helps prevent heart disease and cancer) and magnesium (strengthens bones).

- *Brazil Nuts*: A 1oz (28g) serving is about eight nuts with 4g protein, 190 calories, and 7g monosaturated fat. Brazil nuts are packed with selenium (an antioxidant) and phosphorus (strengthens bones and teeth, and assists with energy metabolism).

---

2   The FDA statement can be found here: www.fda.gov/Food/IngredientsPackagingLabeling/LabelingNutrition/ucm217762.htm.

- *Cashews*: A 1oz (28g) serving is about 18 nuts with 4g protein, 160 calories, and 8g monosaturated fat. Cashews are rich in selenium, magnesium, phosphorus, and iron.

- *Hazelnuts*: A 1oz (28g) serving is about 20 nuts with 4g protein, 180 calories, and 3g monosaturated fat. Hazelnuts contain large amounts of Vitamin E.

- *Macadamias*: A 1oz (28g) serving is about 12 nuts with 2g protein, 200 calories, and 17g monosaturated fat. Macadamias have the highest level of unsaturated fat (cholesterol lowering).

- *Peanuts*: (not actually a nut, but a legume, though often thought of as a nut so here it is!) A 1oz (28g) serving is about 28 nuts with 7g protein, 170 calories, and 7g monosaturated fat. Peanuts are a good source of Vitamin B3 (promoting healthy skin), Vitamin E and zinc (renewing tissue), potassium (good for muscles), and Vitamin B6 (boosts immunity). Can be an allergen.

- *Pecans*: A 1oz (28g) serving is about 20 halves with 3g protein, 200 calories, and 12g monosaturated fat. Pecans are packed with Vitamin B1 (provides thiamine energy) and zinc.

- *Pistachios*: A 1oz (28g) serving is about 45 nuts with 6g protein, 160 calories, and 7g monosaturated fat. Pistachios are full of phosphorus, which is the second most important element, after calcium, for maintaining healthy bones.

- *Walnuts*: A 1oz (28g) serving is about 14 halves with 4g protein, 190 calories, and 2.5g monosaturated fat. Walnuts have the highest amount of Omega-3s (reducing fat and cholesterol). Chinese medicine praises walnuts as "brain food." Their high Omega-3 content alone would account for this, but also because they have the "doctrine of signature" (see Chapter 4): they look like a human brain. For all of these reasons, walnuts are my favorite nut.

HERBS FOR WINTER

A long, cold winter will wear down the body and dull the mind. Some herbs can give us a bit of a boost that enlivens the season without redirecting the Ultimate Yin. The following tonic herbs must be used with caution and only after obtaining professional advice from a qualified herbalist:

- *He shou wu (Polygonum multiflorum)*: This herb has become famous for allegedly turning grey hair back to black. Maybe? It definitely works well as a Liver blood and Kidney essence tonic for conditions of premature ejaculation, lower body weakness, blurred vision, and signs of premature aging. It is often combined with *dang gui* and/or *ren Shen*.

- *Dong chong xia cao* (better known by the English name Cordyceps): This fungus grows on caterpillars and, however shocking that may seem, has been used by Chinese (and other) athletes for its proven ability to boost stamina and speed recovery from physical stress. It is also good for recovering from a long illness.

- *Huang Qi (Astragalus membranaceus)*: This is one of my favorite herbs because it acts like a gentle version of ginseng, which is often too harsh for most common conditions, to invigorate the body's overall qi status. *Huang Qi* tonifies the Spleen, Lungs, and Kidneys to augment the Defensive Qi against pathogens, and improve food absorption and generalized debility.

RECIPES FOR WINTER

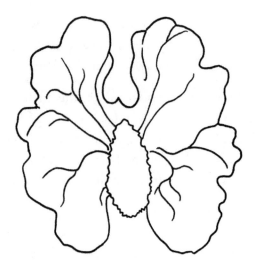

Fruit and Nut Truffles

(Makes about 36 1-inch truffles)

Dried fruit—the yin condition of a yang food—combined with nuts and fragrant spices, makes a wonderfully healthy dessert or snack. Much better than way-too-sweet fudge for winter holidays.

1 cup pitted dates

1 cup unsulfured dried apricots

½ cup dried cranberries, dried cherries, or raisins

1 cup water

1½ tsp grated orange zest

1½ tsp grated lemon zest

1½ tbsp lemon juice

½ cup ground toasted walnuts

½ cup ground toasted almonds (or use different varieties of nuts)

1 tsp cinnamon

3 tbsp unsweetened cocoa powder

2 tbsp confectioners' sugar, sifted

¾ cup toasted unsweetened shredded coconut

Put the dates, dried apricots, dried cranberries, and water in a saucepan, cover, bring to the boil and simmer on medium-low heat until the fruit has softened—about 10 minutes.

Drain the fruit, reserving the liquid. Purée the cooked fruit in food processor, adding only as much of the reserved liquid as is needed to make a smooth, thick paste.

In a mixing bowl, combine the orange zest, lemon zest, and lemon juice. Add the puréed fruit and walnuts, almonds, cinnamon, cocoa, and sugar, and mix well. Taking a teaspoon at a time, form the fruit and nut mixture into balls about an inch in diameter. Roll each ball in the coconut and arrange in a single layer on a serving platter.

Chill for at least 20 minutes before serving. Longer chilling gives a deeper flavor and firmer truffles. This will keep for up to three weeks in sealed container in the refrigerator. If stacked, put wax paper between the layers.

Moroccan Stew

(Serves 6–8)

The fragrance of this dish is almost reason enough to make it. Combine these warming spices with the nuttiness of the garbanzo (chick pea) bean and you have a delicious way to enjoy this ancient food that originated in the Middle East about 5000 years ago. Rich in protein, calcium, iron, and the B vitamins, the garbanzo bean is one of the most nutritious members of the legume family and is naturally suited to the winter diet. The *Jing* contained within its durable structure is a perfect food for this season.

This bean needs to be soaked for a long time—overnight is good. A ¾ cup of dried garbanzos will yield about 1½ cups of cooked beans. You can also find organic canned beans in a good food market.

3 cups coarsely chopped onions	½ tsp paprika
½ cup olive oil	1 cup sliced carrots
2 cloves garlic, minced	4 cups cubed sweet potatoes
1 tsp ground cumin	1 green pepper, sliced in strips
1 tsp turmeric	4 cups sliced zucchini
½ tsp cinnamon	3 cups cubed eggplant
¼–1 tsp cayenne	

2 fresh tomatoes chopped, or a 28oz (800g) can

1½ cups cooked garbanzo beans, or a 5oz (400g) can

¾ cup raisins

¼ cup chopped fresh parsley

In a large soup pot, sauté the onions in the oil for a few minutes. Add the garlic and the spices, stirring constantly for about two minutes (the temperature should not be too hot). Add the carrots and stir for two minutes, then the potatoes for two minutes, then add the pepper, the zucchini, and finally the eggplant. Stir in the tomatoes, then the garbanzos and raisins. You may want to add a little liquid: water or tomato juice. Cover the pot and simmer over a low heat until all the vegetables are tender—about 30 minutes.

Garnish with parsley just before serving.

SPIRIT RETURNS TO EARTH

The process of spiritual awakening, as presented in this book, may take place as a continuous unfolding of your basic goodness. However, there isn't a final enlightenment, at least not as long as we live in the Five Phases. The great Dao began the evolution of matter some 14 billion years ago and, as far as we know, human beings exist as the highest earthly form of substance unfolding toward pure consciousness. This progress was mapped out a thousand years ago when a Daoist sage said, "Transform essence into energy, refine energy into Spirit, awaken Spirit and return to the Dao." This returning has many roads.

Of all the countless possibilities for the future of life on earth, two stand in stark contrast to one another. Our current condition of global delusion has led to sweeping environmental degradation, gross inhumanity, weapons of ultimate destruction, lack of visionary leadership, and overwhelming greed. If this continues, it may finally, perhaps quite suddenly, lead to the extinction of the human species. Alternatively, we may choose the path of spiritual awakening travelled by those who strive to create a healthy environment, ample food, and safe shelter for all of earth's inhabitants so they may live peacefully within the Five Phase Networks and fully share the human potential for benevolence and global goodwill.

But evolution never stops. A third and more rarefied transformation of matter into energy, one that may not happen for millennia, entails the evolution of the body, which is now bound within the Five Phases, into an incarnation of clarified mind awareness dwelling beyond duality of good and bad in the Void of immortality; there would be no attachment to manifestations of life on earth as we know it in present time. That possibility, fantastic as it seems, presents another version of returning to the Void, a place in which the human species exists only as the mind of Wuji.

However, because we currently live in the stream of the Five Phases on this lovely planet, we should consciously and completely participate in the marvelous seasonal cycle that includes family, friends, careers, fulfilments, and dreams—all the wonderful flesh and blood attachments to life on earth. At this level of spiritual awakening we can personify the virtue of basic goodness, develop our energy, and refine our mind for the admirable purpose of becoming a more compassionate and cheerful person. We do this hoping not only to have better health but also to return to the state of well-being when we had no animosity, prejudice, greed, or deep dissatisfactions of mind. Our continual recycling of essence, energy, and Spirit—through qigong and mediation practice—makes our shared earth a positive and joyous environment for the evolution of humankind. Once again, the Yellow Emperor has shown us the path.

> Health and well-being can only be achieved by
> Remaining centered with one's spirit,
> Guarding against squandering one's energy,
> Maintaining the constant flow of qi and blood,
> Adapting to the changing seasonal influences,
> And nourishing oneself by cultivating
> a tranquil heart and mind.
>
> (*The Yellow Emperor's Classic of Medicine*)

REFERENCES

Bateson, G. (1979) *Mind and Nature*. New York: Bantam Press.

Becker, R. and Selden, G. (1985) *The Body Electric: Electromagnetism and the Foundation of Life*. New York: William Morrow.

Beinfield, H. and Korngold, E. (1991) *Between Heaven and Earth: A Guide to Chinese Medicine*. New York: Ballantine Books.

Cohen, K. (1997) *The Way of Qigong: The Art and Science of Chinese Energy Healing*. New York: Ballantine Books.

Flaws, B. (1994) *Imperial Secrets of Health and Longevity*. Boulder, CO: Blue Poppy Press.

Flaws, B. (2010) *Statements of Fact in Traditional Chinese Medicine*. Boulder, CO: Blue Poppy Press.

Foster, R. and Kreitzman, L. (2004) *Rhythms of Life*. New Haven, CT: Yale University Press.

Heisenberg, W. (1971) *Physics and Beyond*. New York: Harper and Row.

Heller, M. (2011) *The DASH Diet Action Plan: Proven to Boost Weight Loss and Improve Health*. New York: Grand Central Publishing.

Hicks, A., Hicks, J., and Mole, P. (2004) *Five Element Constitutional Acupuncture*. London: Churchhill Livingston.

Jiao, G. (1990) *Qigong Essentials For Health Promotion*. China: China Today Press.

Larre, C. and Rochat de la Vallée, E. (1996) *The Seven Emotions: Psychology and Health in Ancient China*. Cambridge: Monkey Press.

Kaptchuk, T. (2000) *The Web That Has No Weaver: Understanding Chinese Medicine*. Chicago, IL: Contemporary Books.

Liu, Z. (2008) *A Study Of Daoist Acupuncture*. Boulder, CO: Blue Poppy Press.

McManus, K., Antinoro, L., and Sacks, F. (2001) "A randomized controlled trial of a moderate-fat, low-energy diet compared with a low-fat, low-energy diet for weight loss in overweight adults." *International Journal of Obesity 25*, 10, 1503–1511.

Maciocia, G. (2009) *The Psyche in Chinese Medicine*. London: Churchhill Livingston.

Manaka, T., Itaya, K., and Birch, S. (1995) *Chasing The Dragon's Tail*. Brookline, MA: Paradigm.

Matsumoto, K. and Birch, S. (1988) *Hara Diagnosis: Reflections on the Sea.* Brookline, MA: Paradigm Books.

Needham, J. (1978) *Science and Civilization in China.* Cambridge: Cambridge University Press.

Ni, M. (1995) *The Yellow Emperor's Classic of Medicine.* Boston, MA: Shambhala.

O'Connor, J. and Bensky, D. (eds) (1985) *Acupuncture: A Comprehensive Text.* Seattle, WA: Eastland Press.

Oldstone-Moore, J. (2003) *Taoism.* New York: Oxford University Press.

Schuessler, A. (2007) *ABC Etymological Dictionary of Old Chinese.* Honolulu, HI: University of Hawaii Press.

Sivin, N. (1987) *Traditional Medicine in Contemporary China.* Ann Arbor, MI: University of Michigan, Center for Chinese Studies.

Tianjun, L. and Chen, K. (eds) (2010) *Chinese Medical Qigong.* London: Jessica Kingsley Publishers.

Unschuld, P. (2003) *Huang Di Nei Jing Su Wen: Nature, Knowledge, Imagery in an Ancient Chinese Medical Text.* Berkeley, CA: University of California Press.

Watson, B. (1996) *Chuang Tzu.* New York: Columbia University Press.

Wong, E. (1992) *Cultivating Stillness.* Boston, MA: Shambhala.

Wong, E. (2000) *The Tao of Health, Longevity, and Immortality.* Boston, MA: Shambhala.

Suggested Reading

Blofeld, J. (1985) *Taoism The Road To Immortality*. Boston, MA: Shambhala.

Hinton, D. (2013) *The Four Chinese Classics*. Berkeley, CA: Counterpoint.

Jahnke, R. (2002) *The Healing Promise Of Qi*. Chicago, IL: Contemporary Books.

Kohn, L. (ed) (1989) *Taoist Meditation And Longevity Techniques*. Ann Arbor, MI: University of Michigan.

Mitchell, D. (2011) *Daoist Nei Gong*. London: Singing Dragon.

Pine, R. (1996) *Lao-tzu's Taoteching*. San Francisco, CA: Mercury House.

Pitchford, P. (2002) *Healing With Whole Foods*. Berkeley, CA: North Atlantic Books.

Robinet, I. (1993) *Taoist Meditation*. Albany, NY: State University of New York Press.

Watts, A. (1998) *Taoism Way Beyond Seeking*, Boston, MA: Tuttle Publishing.

Wong, E. (1997) *The Shambhala Guide To Taoism*. Boston, MA: Shambhala.

Wu, Z. (2006) *Vital Breath Of The Dao*. St. Paul, MN: Dragon Door Publications.

INDEX